Just
a
NURSE

Just a Nurse

2024 YGTMedia Co. Press Trade Paperback Edition.

Published in Canada, for Global Distribution by YGTMedia Co.
www.ygtmedia.co
For more information email: info@ygtmedia.co

ISBN trade paperback: 978-1-998754-69-4
eBook: 978-1-998754-70-0

To order additional copies of this book:
info@ygtmedia.co

COVER PHOTO: Noelle Smith

Just
a
NURSE

MEMOIR ON THE
HEARTBEAT OF HEALING

ASHLEY CHANCELLOR, RN

Table of Contents

Dedication

This book is dedicated to every nurse out there who feels too tired to keep going; to every first responder who feels like they haven't had a moment to breathe without a mask; to the health-care worker who feels lost and broken—endlessly stuck in a system that relies on the bedside staff as its very own beating heart, yet cannot care for us enough to give us a break. To each of us who has been depleted by a system that has left us feeling war torn when all we have ever wanted to do is love and help. I see you. I am you. I am here for you.

Introduction

Everyone knows a nurse, teacher, or first responder. Someone who cares about other people, placing their needs behind those of others. We all recognize the strength and courage it takes for our heroes to serve and protect, respond to emergencies, and meet people in their time of need. But no one knows what to do when the strong begin to crumble.

In our pain and darkest moments, the most any of us need is someone to sit with us, reminding us of our own abilities to heal the awful wounds we have endured. We need to heal ourselves so we can take better care of each other.

Time, kindness, and a sprinkle of laughter can and will improve our lives and the world at large. You don't have to take my advice, though, as I'm just a nurse.

Through my nursing travels you'll see the good, the bad, and the honest. In these pages lie the heartbreaks and tears that accompany the inevitable callousness that hardens one's edges from a job we give our hearts to. This is the journey of a nurse who loved so much it broke her into a thousand jagged pieces; a nurse whose passion for the field destroyed not only her body but also her heart and mind; a nurse determined to heal herself despite the system that damaged her so brutally.

I'm not aware of many other career paths that ask, "*Why* did you get into this field?" quite as often as nursing. The self-introductions most first days of school held allowed us to clearly see the different backgrounds of us all. Little did we know we'd be spending some of the most frustrating and trying hours together in study groups and at patient bedsides frantically absorbing every piece of knowledge thrown our way. We were eager and fearful of the day when someone's life would sit delicately in our hands and we would have the knowledge and know-how to save it. Such sobering fears fueled the intensity and drive on our journey to becoming registered nurses.

Many people make their way into nursing after experiencing a traumatic event, finding inspiration in the staff who provided great care. Others come from nursing families, anxious to write RN after their name and knowing firsthand the road that lies ahead leads to a field that quite literally becomes one's identity. Others still are logistic students who see nursing as an entryway to higher-degreed positions, and some come from outlying health-care fields looking for purpose in the ways nursing offers.

Not many people grow up dreaming of the selfless lifestyle required to work night shifts, weekends, and holiday requirements, not to mention on-call schedules and the intense physical and emotional demands of a life spent responding to people in their greatest times of need. Nursing is a field that requires you to put your own needs, biases, and emotions on a shelf in exchange for helping a stranger.

Every new semester, clinical assignment, and class brought an opportunity for introductions and the retelling of our *why*, a ritual that constantly reminded us of our dedication to and reasoning for making all the long hours, hard work, and stress worth it. Most of us were there to make some positive impact on the world in whatever way we could. Nursing has a type of calling on one's life. It seems to choose a person to answer the need to help others in their weakest moments.

Doctors have been glorified by popular television shows like *Grey's Anatomy*, *ER*, and *Scrubs*. They've been pictured as the friendly face for the patient, the ones pulling all-nighters, the specialists staring at heart rhythms and calling a Code Blue to notify CPR teams to save a life at the brink of death. What viewers don't realize, however, is that those actors are playing out scenes oftentimes handled by the nursing staff who stand tirelessly at patients' bedsides. Nurses are the eyes and ears for the patients and the physicians; they are dedicated to advocating for people in need while providing quality care.

Living by the oath to "do no harm" and known as the "backbone of health care," nurses are the very foundation of a system that relies on them to provide compassionate and safe care. Patients put their hope and trust into the hands of willing nurses to manage their well-being at a time when they are most vulnerable. No wonder nursing has been voted the most trusted profession in American society for more than twenty years.

Registered nurses are not the only ones working intimately at patient bedsides, and they're not the only ones feeling the strain of burnout. Among the few caring physicians left at bedside, respiratory therapists and nursing assistants are undoubtedly some of the most under-recognized caregivers dedicated to patients. Thus, it's not just nurses feeling the negative effects of a system that so obviously places profits before patients. To those working alongside us, I see your footsteps the same as my own. You have not been forgotten. The terms *nurse* and *nursing* within these pages include you as well. We would be nowhere without our literal heart and lungs.

This story is not unlike those of other nurses who have felt the effects of burnout, no longer able to care for others or themselves—no longer fueled by their *why*. I hope you can see yourself in these pages; I hope you can bite your lip to get through the rough stories, let yourself cry when the tears come, and feel like you're laughing next to me in scrubs during the traumatic parts.

My *why* for nursing has never changed: I still want to help people. Unfortunately, it took completely losing myself in the care of others to learn to help myself first. I hope you see that *you*—just as much as our patients—deserve the love and compassion you give, and that you learn to love yourself before sacrificing for others.

1. Emergency Laughter
May 2008

I stood in the entry to the trauma room in the emergency department (ER). There were a dozen staff rushing around one patient. Each life saver, dressed in light blue scrubs, seemed to be doing their own task yet was simultaneously working with everyone like all parts of an engine firing at precisely the right time.

Gasp! How cool that I am getting to witness a real-live trauma brought in.

The emergency medical technicians (EMTs), dressed in black uniforms, efficiently navigated the winding halls of the ER, then whipped the gurney into the trauma bay as if they had done it a million times. They aligned the gurney perfectly with the hospital bed, then the sound of brakes locking into place echoed above the chaos occurring around the room. Some nurses were getting cables ready, while other nurses rushed in to put on gloves to help with the transfer. The EMTs rambled off facts about age, gender, and injuries: "Twenty-three-year-old female, passenger in a motor vehicle accident . . ."

I was speechless. There I was, standing in the corner of the room in pristine all-white scrubs, wearing minimal makeup and a watch with a second hand. A periwinkle stethoscope was draped around my neck waiting to be used, but I was only playing dress-up.

This was the only day I'd get to experience an ER, a feat my clinical instructor pulled off on her own. I'd thought when going into nursing school there would be perfectly planned clinicals with time afterward for reflection, chances to learn and be hands on, and adequate time to decide what specialty I might prefer. But alas, neither program I attended seemed to offer every experience one could want.

My instructor had worked at this large trauma hospital for years and was well known. She was also someone who wasn't afraid to ask for things. She was the kind of nurse I hoped to be one day: a well-experienced one who could handle any situation and had lots of friends within the system.

As a young nursing student, I had longed for the day when I could confidently respond to someone in need and make a difference in their life. It was a yearning that became an obsession when the instructor arrived two hours late one day, her lab coat covered in blood after stopping at an accident on her way in. I remember peppering her with questions about what she did and how she knew to do it.

"You learn to keep calm and focus on the basics. Which are . . . ?"

"Airway, breathing, circulation!" my classmates and I shouted with excitement and pleasure for knowing the answer. We fed off the teaching moment in the presence of a real-life angel who was holding the severed leg of a stranger met just minutes prior, petrified of the day we might be in the same (un)fortunate moment and would need to respond.

Over lunch the instructor explained the Good Samaritan Law and our obligation, once licensed, to respond to emergencies at all times. I was in awe, though that moment seemed like a distant possibility and eons of experience away seeing as how I didn't even yet know how to put IVs in, let alone save a life.

The instructor had managed to arrange a day for each of her students to shadow in the ER while the other students spent their day on the medical floor giving bed baths, reviewing medications, and trying not to reveal to every patient we were brand new, terrified about harming them, and absolutely clueless about how to adequately care for people.

When it was my day in the ER, I got to witness a well-organized team respond to a crisis. It was beautifully compelling to watch a team of people work diligently to save the life of someone they didn't know. I tucked back the wave of emotion creeping up my throat. I was proud and excited to be entering this amazing field but also hugely sad for the young woman lying on the stretcher.

I watched as her limp body was hoisted from the gurney to the stretcher on an efficient count: "One, two, three!" Everyone in the room took this as the starting point for quickly carrying out their individual tasks while the EMTs continued answering questions and rattling off vital signs and heart rhythms.

"Twenty-three-year-old female, passenger side, driver died on impact. It was her boyfriend. Apparently, they were just a block away from home when they were T-boned at a four-way. Infant at home. Parents of the girl are on their way in."

My heart ached as the voice in my head shouted, "Move faster! Didn't you hear?! She has a baby at home and people who love her! She could have died too. She needs help! HELP HER!" I wanted to jump in, to help in any way I could, but I didn't have a clue what to do except stand in the spot I'd been told to stay in, out of the way and watching. Watching helplessly. Then, in unison, the team turned the patient on her side to cut off her clothes.

"Slippery Rock?! Nope, you gotta take her somewhere else," Joe, the nurse I had been assigned to shadow, said with a chuckle as he cut through the back of the black hoodie, dividing the neon green letters with each snip of the trauma shears. The other nurses started laughing as they all poked fun at the local State school known for its partying students.

"We're all full," Joe said, continuing his joking with the EMTs. "No room for Slippery Rock alumni here." Laughter ensued, and the EMTs replied that they needed a coffee break and didn't have time to take her anywhere else. Rage coursed through my body.

WHAT ARE YOU PEOPLE TALKING ABOUT?! This is a young woman whose world has forever changed for the worse, and you have the nerve to poke fun? It took everything inside me to remain in my designated spot. I wanted to jump in and take over, to care for her soul, to rewind the clock, and to change the intersection!

The team moved efficiently, placing IVs, collecting blood, cleaning wounds, and calling out assessments about pupils and reflexes. Blood-soaked clothing and gauze covered the floor as I stood back taking it all in, consumed by awe and envy over wanting to be that well-oiled kind of nurse someday.

With one more laugh and a jovial "Sayonara," the EMTs exited the room. The side rails locked into place with the release of the bed wheels, then the team was ready to move. Standing over the freshly draped patient was a gray-scrub-clad person holding a football-sized clear bag connected to the tube inside the young woman's mouth. I saw her chest rise with every squeeze of the bag. *This is manual ventilation*, I thought as lecture terms clicked with real-life events. *That must be a respiratory therapist*, I realized, connecting the dots to the person squeezing the plastic football.

"Want to go to MRI?" Joe asked me with a smile while nodding toward the door. He knew I'd never pass up this experience as a nursing student. Of course, I wanted to go to MRI! I wanted to see the inside of an MRI room, to watch every living moment of what was happening, to learn what they were scanning for, to hear people talk in a language I was still learning to understand. I wanted to do it all! I grabbed both sides of my stethoscope as if putting on a backpack and kept up with the fast pace of the team.

We rounded corners while Joe shouted, "STAT MRI coming through!" to make room for the gurney rushing by. Just then, my instructor popped out from behind one of the corners and said it was time for lunch. Relief washed over me, then sadness. I wasn't done with this patient. I needed to go with her; I needed to find out everything about her journey. But my inability to offer any real help as a student nurse flashed in my mind, so I nodded and then turned to Joe as I stepped away from the stretcher.

"Glad you got to see that! Maybe we'll see you in the ER one day!" Joe said cheerfully without stopping.

As I obediently followed my instructor to the cafeteria, she questioned me about the experience and asked what I got to see. I gave her the short version, the parts my other classmates would be excited about—the trauma, the accident, the meds I recognized when they were called out. I knew my classmates would be envious of this experience and yet all I wanted to do was march back there and tell them they should be more focused on the job and less focused on laughing and telling stories. I didn't understand how people could be so lighthearted in a moment of tragedy. Yes, they were saving her life and she was a priority hospital-wide, but I just didn't get why they laughed so much.

At lunch, I opened up to my teacher about the joking. I used the word *insensitive* to describe their behavior. I vowed right then to not be one of those insensitive nurses one day. I was going to be different.

"I know it seems cold-hearted from the outside, but laughter can relieve the heaviness and allows the team to continue working. Trust me, everyone in that room was feeling what you were feeling and understood the severity of the situation; they've just toughened up to the emotional side."

My heart hurt. *Would I get to be that tough one day?*

2. Trauma Warning
April 1987 – May 2003

It is estimated that more than 60 percent of health-care workers have experienced a form of childhood trauma.

At seven years old, standing on the steps of our local church, I coached my mother through a manic-depressive episode and out of killing herself. It's my first memory of feeling someone else's pain and having the desire to make them better. It was also the first of many occasions I would stop a family member from taking their own life. At much too young of an age, I was exposed to a world engulfed in mental health issues, violence, and addiction. The adults in my life navigated their own lost childhoods and the stress of poverty, while I worried about my safety and future as well as the safety and future of my two younger siblings.

When I was ten, we moved from a basement apartment in the ghettos of Pittsburgh to my grandparents' pink Victorian house in the suburbs. My world suddenly flipped on its head. Walking to the foodbank and learning to go without turned into sit-down dinners at a table and a bed of my own. It was a dramatic change, to say the least.

Patience and empathy were not traits that came naturally to either of my grandparents, nor were they shy about their disdain for having children interrupt their retirement. We learned to tiptoe around volatile emotions, just happy to have a roof over our heads and some kind of structure. There were plenty of harsh words plus high expectations—and with no support as to how to reach them. I learned my grandparents seemed to be more tolerant of my existence when I was contributing, so I jumped when they said jump and fell in line with the new routines as best I could.

By the time we had moved in, my step-grandmother was on her second open-heart surgery. She was a "frequent flier" at the hospitals, requiring recurrent overnight stays to treat her multitude of ailments. It became part of our routine to visit her, take her overnight bag, then adjust to her new discharge routines. Sickness wasn't something she was ashamed of but rather something she took pride in; she wore each surgery and medical diagnosis like a badge of honor. She didn't tolerate anyone else around her feeling unwell or stealing her attention, and she certainly didn't like it when the doctors told her to quit smoking.

Standing at a whopping four feet and eleven inches, she had the ability to make everyone feel smaller than she was. It was a special talent. Rather than argue with her, I learned to stay on her good side by opening pill bottles and dressing wounds slow to heal.

My grandfather died the summer before my senior year. Unlike my step-grandmother, he was a fastidious atheist who staunchly believed there was nothing beyond life here on earth. He despised doting or any attention that made him appear weak, as he always prided himself on being strong and healthy.

At first, he seemed to defy the grim odds the doctors had given him with his cancer diagnosis. He continued to drive and manage home repairs. Over the period of just a few weeks, however, I watched this unbreakable strength wither into a helpless, frail old man. I spent the short time leading up to his passing helping him around the house and being his eyes so he could keep driving. He didn't need his hand held or wounds bandaged, he needed someone to ensure his independence until the very end.

Caregiving seemed to be in my DNA, something innate that just wanted everyone to be free of pain and have their needs met. I understood what it felt like to be broken and forgotten. I took on the role of sitting with people in their pain and discomfort long before becoming a nurse.

3. Medicine
May 2003

To be honest, I didn't realize I was uncomfortable until I was sitting in class. Because I was still actively participating on the dance team, it was a shock to everyone that I, a fifteen-year-old, had back pain. The ache ran down both legs and radiated through my hips, making my toes numb. I couldn't focus on learning; the only thing gnawing at my brain was the excruciating pain. It took months of working our way through specialists and tests before I was diagnosed with a herniated disc. Scans revealed the injury was old and had begun healing. Surgery was an option, but the conservative neurosurgeon wanted to start with physical therapy instead.

Pain has a way of wearing down one's spirit. Hoping for immediate relief, I wanted narcotics. My step-grandmother took high-dose pain relievers after various procedures, her pain and anger seemingly washed away by Western medicine. I also thought it would be cool to tell my friends I was on prescribed medications, like it made my injury more real somehow.

Fortunately, the doctor prescribed me naproxen. He explained it was a high-dose anti-inflammatory, like a beefed-up ibuprofen. I was also to start weekly physical therapy sessions with the hope of avoiding surgery. I felt important. I felt I had a reason for people to finally care about me. There was something actually wrong and I was seeing a doctor for it—certainly this would make me matter, right?

Going to physical therapy (PT) was self-driven. I had to make my own appointments and walk to the clinic after school. I didn't mind, though. I enjoyed the office; it looked like an adult day care with its treadmills and brightly colored yoga balls, bands, and ramps in every corner. The naproxen improved my pain enough so I could sit through class, but it was the PT, chiropractic adjustments, and massage therapy that started to *fix* the injury. The muscles in my back and hips were chronically tight, and my being stretched and worked out regularly helped the discomfort as well as my posture and strength in dance.

I was slowly feeling better, and by the time I had completed eight weeks of PT, I had secured an internship at the clinic. I sat with patients and helped them count their reps, folded towels, and made sure the hot packs had enough water. I was also permitted to remove the electrodes from the patients and escort them to their next activity. It was fun. I enjoyed visiting with the patients and hearing about how they acquired their knee replacement, the shoulder injury from years of playing tennis, or how they lost fine motor skills after experiencing a stroke. It was a space of recovery, and new opportunities waited on the other side. It inspired me to want to help people I didn't know. I imagine this is where the glowing embers for becoming a doctor one day were ignited.

4. Nursing School Dreams
March 2004 – December 2010

As a little girl I used to have a speech about how I wanted to be a teacher on Mondays, a lawyer on Tuesdays, a doctor on Wednesdays, a truck driver on Thursdays, and then back in town by Sunday to preach in church. Oh my, was I ambitious!

My autobiography circa 1999, a sixth-grade class project, featured a two-page hand-drawn centerfold of a courtroom and a chapter dedicated to my ambition for upholding the law. I did not have the funding, academics, or the discipline to pursue such a lofty goal, but when the guidance counselor sat me down and told me I was eligible for a career apprenticeship and asked what field I wanted to study, I responded with a very matter-of-fact answer: "I want to be a doctor." We were both surprised.

The apprenticeship was for a nursing position, not to shadow a doctor. I knew doctors and nurses worked side by side, and as long as I could experience what life was like from the provider side, I knew it would be beneficial. After writing an essay on why I should be chosen and purchasing scrubs in an adult large when a small would have sufficed, I rode two city buses across town in my new oversized attire to shadow a nurse.

It didn't take long for me to realize that everything I admired about being a doctor—comforting patients, listening to lungs, giving medications, starting IVs, the real conduction of patient care—was actually done by a nurse. I watched in admiration while the nurses confidently managed the care of six patients, all with various ailments and needs. The efficiency with which they performed tasks and left patients feeling comforted and taken care of struck me in the heart. Meanwhile, I watched as doctors rushed in and out, careful not to bond with patients.

In chatting with the nurses, I learned many of them had attended local diploma programs and were paying off their school debt while working on the floor. My future suddenly seemed attainable. I was exactly where I needed to be.

I applied for a diploma program and to my own surprise tested high enough to get in. On the first day, the students had their egos stroked by the welcoming committee who proclaimed us "the cream of the crop." You could feel the confidence in the air, although I felt inadequate when they acknowledged many people in the room had master's degrees. We, the high school graduates, were met with: "You're probably used to getting As," to which we all nodded in agreement. Except I wasn't an "A" student. I knew I was capable of it, but I had an inability to focus and no discipline at home to do homework. I skirted through high school as a C student, and I was hopeful to learn the study skills in nursing school I so desperately lacked at home.

There was a general feeling of confidence in the room that encouraged me to believe in myself. Then, without hesitation, our welcome speech turned into a warning: "All of you will struggle in this program." *Gulp.* The comment seemed taunting, even eerie, as if to tread lightly if a nursing career was what you truly wanted. The program was cutthroat with a high bar of expectation, and it was not afraid to shatter our dreams.

Our main classroom was on the ground floor of an office building and was not how I'd pictured any kind of college. The dreams of staying in a dormitory and making friends my own age were replaced by the reality of a rundown, lonely apartment and two long bus rides to school on the other side of town. I worked three part-time jobs while navigating nursing school and learning how to be on my own.

One day the instructor stood at the front of the classroom next to her projector, clicking through slides and presenting on community health nursing. The pictures were devastating and heartbreaking. Hurricane Katrina had destroyed the Gulf Coast of the US the year prior. More than 74,000 volunteers responded to help the 160,000 people in need of resources, first aid, and compassion. I was awed by every story she shared about her volunteer time spent saving the lives of people in absolute critical need.

The pictures showed people connected to IV poles, with bandaged wounds and lost hope, lying in makeshift medical wards in shopping malls and stadiums. The instructor told us about the working conditions and lack of supplies. She spoke of her long days that turned into nights that turned back into days, all while she wore the same pair of scrubs. Each story she recalled sent us through a roller coaster of emotions as we listened intently to ones about survival and love and human compassion and tragedy. And then there was the medical terminology that was beyond our baby nursing minds. She put names to faces and concluded the presentation with pictures of earlier patients now looking healthier and stronger with smiles on their faces. I was terrified. I was inspired. *That's the kind of nurse I want to be one day. I want to be able to respond and make a difference.* I wanted to be just like the hero standing in front of our classroom.

I excelled in clinicals, quickly mastering hands-on techniques and caring for patients. But I struggled with classwork. Coordinating school with clinicals, studying, and working my numerous part-time jobs was becoming unfeasible. Then the dam broke after nine months of an impossible balancing act—I failed Pharmacy and would need to retake it in night school. The fast-paced diploma program I'd lucked my way into had high expectations and left little room for error. It took me another nine months to learn that one test question could, in fact, impact your future. I failed Adult Cardiac Nursing, earning just shy of 76 percent (the mandatory grade for passing), and I was let go from the program six weeks before graduation.

Swallowing my pride and admitting failure was devastating, but I only had a few weeks before the local community college closed fall enrollment, so there was no time for tears. I rushed through entry exams and student interviews in desperation to secure a seat, sure to become a nurse eventually.

The second time through didn't make the program any easier other than my being privy to the obstacle course that lay ahead. I enjoyed the relief offered by the required electives, finding interest and an easy A in the likes of Yoga and Pottery. When it came to nursing courses, I kept my head down and focused on the day when I would eventually be responsible for my own patients.

The thrill of writing RN at the end of my name was my holy grail. To be legally granted the right to sign my name and proudly claim the title of Registered Nurse is one that warrants balloons. Nurses live for the letters after their names, wearing each certification and specialty mastered like a badge of honor. We're taught our signature means something: it can positively affect lives and bears power like a superhero cape, and the letters after it are proof of the hard work we've put in.

Making a positive impact on lives is sure reason enough for every nurse I know to look forward to earning their RN designation. But those initials become bigger than the person they're attached to when someone finds themselves lost in the care of others. Or at least that's what happened to me.

5. An Environment of Mercy
September 2010

Before I knew it, I was being assigned my senior semester externship. The program arranged for each student to spend eight weeks working the schedule of an orienting (precepting) nurse at various hospitals in town. The opportunity offered real-life, hands-on nursing experience before we headed out as new grads, a feat none of us felt ready for.

I had no clue what kind of hospital I wanted to work in . . . Something busy with an ICU and serious injuries? But that was most hospitals it seemed. I longed to make a difference in a place where there was high trauma and big impact. However, I would take any assignment I was offered.

Coming out of the 2008 recession, we students were constantly being reminded that hospitals were on hiring freezes and it would be difficult to find jobs as new nurses. We therefore breathed in hope as we waited for our senior assignments, as these apprenticeships could possibly lead to job offers. On the day of the announcements, anticipation grew in the room. Everyone was squirming from the reality of becoming real nurses.

"Ashley Chancellor, Burn ICU." *Burn ICU?! I can't do that!* I gulped back my lunch.

Vivid memories began flashing through my mind of the short walk we had taken through the burn unit. During the tour past ICU beds filled with patients wrapped in gauze, we paused in the treatment room encircling two metal tables. The tables were unique to treating burn patients because they allowed a constant flow of cool liquid to wash away burned tissue as it was scraped from the patients' bodies. We'd stood in this room a little longer than I was comfortable with, discussing the massive doses of pain medication used for these patients and reviewing body percentage calcs (calculating drip rates and liters of hydration needed for their cells' extreme loss of hydration).

Although I was training to be a nurse, there were some things I wasn't yet ready to handle. In that walk-through, my stomach turned at the thought of having to treat someone who was screaming out in pain and begging me to stop. My heart couldn't handle that kind of heroism. But my instructor's warning about job opportunities flashed in my brain, and I wanted to be grateful for the potential ICU exposure.

The recitation of the list continued, placing some of my colleagues in ICUs, some on medical floors, and all in various units across the city. I snapped back to reality when Angela's name was called.

"Cardiovascular Intensive Care Unit."

Why couldn't I have something cool like that? I became washed over by worry with the thought of my assignment once again but tried to embrace the fact that I'd have a familiar face at the same hospital at least.

The reading of names concluded and the auditorium erupted with life as people gathered their notebooks and bags with eager anticipation of finding their friends and comparing assignments. Angela slowly stood up next to me, and we both reached for our bags.

"Ashley Chancellor, please see me before you leave," a stern voice called from the front of the auditorium.

"I'm not that excited about CVICU," Angela said with a frown. Angela had always been positive and was one of the gentlest souls I'd ever met. Nursing school friends are like no other. Going through such a grueling program and managing the massive amounts of stress together creates a team mentality that promotes widespread encouragement for everyone to succeed. A sigh of relief washed over me.

"Ugh, I'm not excited either. Burn ICU sounds awful!"

"Are you kidding me?! That sounds so cool! I would love the Burn ICU! Maybe you can introduce me to the manager at some point?"

We both resolved in those short moments to make the most of our placements. If taking the burn apprenticeship meant I could get my friend closer to her dream, then that was my purpose. I didn't know if I could survive eight weeks in such an intense environment, but I would try. I sauntered to the front of the auditorium with my friend at my side.

"Are you okay?" My instructor's genuine concern was clear in the question.

"Yeah, I think so," I responded, unsure of what she was referring to.

"When I read off your assignment, you looked like you might faint."

A thousand worries rushed through my mind. Would I have this opportunity seized from me for my ungratefulness and inability to control my facial expressions? The instructor waited for an answer as my internal battle raged on.

"I . . . I . . . I don't know if I can handle Burn ICU. But I'll take it! I just don't think I'm tough enough for that." I tried not to sound like it wasn't a great opportunity, but she had seen my honest reaction and called me out. I dreaded the thought of having to be on a medical–surgical floor, where nurses are assigned at least five patients. I had seen enough to know I wasn't capable of handling so many patients; I wanted more one-on-one patient care. I pleaded to the empty deity out of habit and to all that was holy that I didn't just lose my opportunity to learn in an ICU.

"You'll be fine," she said with a dismissive tone just before Angela chimed in.

"Miss Thompson! I got assigned the CVICU. Can we switch?"

She paused for a moment, looked back and forth between us and seemed to search for a reason to deny the request. "I don't see why that would be a problem."

Um, pardon? Did you just agree to switch our preceptorships? Did you just say that I don't have to go to the Burn ICU? And not only that but I get to go to the CVICU?! I wanted to jump up and down and hug the stern teacher standing in front of me. I wanted to lift my friend in the air in celebration of her kindness. I beamed ear to ear.

Making a note on her form, the instructor glanced up in annoyance. "Anything else?"

"No. Thank you!" Angela and I chimed in unison, then erupted into giggles and headed for the door before this opportunity could be taken from us. We beamed with enthusiasm and pride for our assignments. We were so excited for our futures and were ready to be the best student nurses we could be.

I learned more in the next two months than I had in what felt like all of nursing school. Most importantly, I learned I had no clue what I was doing. I spent eight weeks bravely jumping in. I attempted my first placements of nasogastric tubes, Foleys (catheters), and most excitingly, IVs. I spent night shifts learning about pathophysiology and waveforms while making note cards of vasopressors and inotropes. I lived, breathed, and absorbed what it would be like to be an actual nurse and responsible for lives.

Nearing the last week of my preceptorship, the unit's spunky, spiky-haired charge nurse offered me a graduate nurse position. I had made it—I was going to be a real nurse!

6. How Good We Had It

February 2011 – September 2013

My first nursing position was at a Catholic hospital located in a part of town not known for its safety. It was a trauma facility bustling with multiple ICUs, a labor and delivery unit, and renowned physicians performing cutting-edge procedures.

Established by nuns in the 1840s, the hospital had become the first training facility in the region. Notwithstanding religious affiliation, race, gender, nationality, or age, the Sisters treated anyone in need of medical services. These women devoted their life to God and thus, found purpose in serving through faith-based care. Midmorning each day, a prayer came over the loudspeaker followed by a moment of silence. There was never a moment for the staff to stop and pray, but hearing it felt like a blessing in and of itself.

At the time, I was a fastidious atheist. I was as sure about the absence of God as I was about the next day being forecast as cloudy. This was Pittsburgh, after all. But I looked forward to the prayer anyway; at least someone was sending hope during these difficult times. A sense of peace lingered after the moment of silence even though the monitors continued to alarm.

Along with the daily prayers, a gentle and short lullaby would be played to announce the birth of each new baby. When things were chaotic and lives were at the brink, hearing those lullabies over the loudspeaker reminded me about the large amounts of beauty and pain each moment of the day held.

What I liked and became spoiled over was the availability of clergy. The Sisters roamed the hospital like resident house cats. Some would bring sweet treats to the staff and share a laugh over a cup of coffee, while others helped roll a patient and change the bedding underneath them. The Sisters came when we called, offered helping hands when they could, and comforted patients and families through dark times. They praised us for the work we were doing and encouraged us through trying shifts. Though I didn't understand their calling, I admired these wonderful women who were there supporting us and our patients.

The unit was staffed with nurses who had worked within the same walls for decades and with the spattering of new grads that seemed to trickle in yearly. The patchwork of staff included senior nurses with more than twenty years' experience who hardly blinked an eye at the things that made us new grads cringe.

The nature of a CVICU brought a steady stream of nomadic nurses to gain experience while chasing bigger dreams of becoming flight nurses, nurse anesthetists, or nurse practitioners. It was a competitive environment that led to in-depth education from the physicians at patient bedsides with a slew of nurses eavesdropping, eager to pick up every shred of medical knowledge and insight we could.

At any given moment there were people trained in Western medicine who could respond to crises even when the doctors stepped off the unit. I dreamed of the day when I would feel as competent as the seasoned nurses I idolized there. It was among these seasoned colleagues who had a passion for caregiving that I learned how to assess patients without the aid of technology, how to monitor for minuscule changes, and how to truly work as a team. They instilled wisdom and a healthy dose of fear into my new grad heart, preparing me for a career that can only be lived and not learned in a book.

"How long before you felt like a real nurse?" I incessantly asked any nurse who had been in the game longer than I had. Though I was gaining knowledge, I still lacked confidence and feared I would never feel fully competent to handle a crisis on my own.

7. Welcome to the Circus
August 2011

"Thank you for choosing us as your emergency medical destination! My name is Stacy, and I will be your nurse for the next thirty minutes." The sing-song tone in which she rattled off these words reminded me of a flight attendant.

Though we were nearing the end of the day, Stacy still looked as fresh as when she arrived in her fitted baby blue scrubs, perfectly curled blonde hair, and chunky silver chain heart necklace. No matter the level of chaos, Stacy and the other seasoned nurses stayed calm, collected, and mostly positive, if only a touch sarcastic.

We were all ready to end the day after nearly twelve hours on our feet, but not before tucking in our latest admission and preparing for the oncoming shift. I had been working in the CVICU as a new nurse for more than six months and was learning the routine fairly well. Then, the comatose patient who had been wheeled in suddenly began sitting up. We all took our spots and held down an appendage as he tried to take a swing at staff and thrashed about in an attempt to get the tube out of his throat. Working in pairs, we applied the blue-and-white wrist restraints gifted to every patient on a breathing machine to limit the patient's ability to hit us.

"Sir, we ask that you keep your arms and legs inside the ride at all times." Stacy's chipper voice continued to sing as if he were listening, but he continued to thrash and fight as we worked to keep him from pulling at anything he could wrap his hands around. Stacy held down his left arm with one hand, while punching the buttons on the IV pump with the other. "Courtesy of our wonderful ER, you have earned yourself a breathing tube—unfortunately, you cannot remove it." Her voice became a little gruff as he tried to push against the team holding him down. "Pam, can you grab some Ativan for this nice man?" she shouted out above the commotion in the room to a team member at the nurses' station. We all giggled at her lighthearted approach to an immensely frustrating situation and egged on her positive demeanor.

This man regularly frequented our ICU to manage the side effects of withdrawal following a lifelong alcohol addiction. He really was quite nice when everything was said and done. He'd always come around after a few days of detoxing in the ICU, appreciative of our care and opening up about his addiction. At discharge we'd wish him well and he'd chuckle that he hoped he wouldn't see us again. But it would only be a matter of weeks before his name would pop up on our admit list again.

Knowing he had good in him kept us all a little more tolerant of his behavior, wishing him well as we discharged him time and time again. Nevertheless, he needed to be tied down and sedated to get through the next forty-eight hours of detoxing. By this point he was trying to sit up again. He kicked out at the nurses and was using every ounce of strength to break through the holds we had on his arms.

We explain to patients that being on a ventilator or breathing machine feels like breathing through a straw. The plastic tube placed into the lungs is connected to a machine that literally breathes for the patient. But the anxiety of having something in your throat, as well as the feeling of suffocation, causes patients to panic, and they instinctively try to dislodge the very tube that is saving their life. It can have detrimental effects to their airway, and it can be life-threatening. In moments of distress it is difficult for patients to understand this, so to manage the anxiety and keep patients safe, we give medications to relax or sedate them for days or weeks while the machine allows their body and lungs to rest.

This patient was clearly panicking. Stacy continued to punch buttons on the pump as Pam charged in with a syringe and alcohol swab. She seamlessly handed the syringe to Stacy, then put both hands on the man's arm, allowing Stacy to "scrub the hub" and inject the medication in the IV.

"Lloyd, stop fighting!" Pam's stern voice demanded without a hint of jest.

"And here we have Pam-the-Ass-Master who will shave your butthole and put glue on it if you keep acting up." We all broke out in cackles at that remark. Even Pam laughed through her tough demeanor.

Soon, the medication began working, causing Lloyd to relax back into the bed. We all moved about each other, tying down appendages, helping secure restraints, taking vital signs, and writing relevant notes on the whiteboard—all the while chatting about anything but the patient less a few terms of assessment needing documenting here and there. We joked about Pam's amazing skills at placing a "butt bag" as we so eloquently called the ostomy bag we secure to someone's backside when they have uncontrollable stooling. Pam could make them leak proof. We then tidied up the room in preparation for the oncoming shift, leaving supplies for tasks still needing completion but that we hadn't had time to do. The next shift began trickling in, putting down their bags and grabbing report sheets.

It hadn't been long since I'd stood clueless in the ER with my blood boiling as I listened to a team ridicule a patient. Yet there I was, jovially caring for this man in crisis. It wasn't that we didn't care—of course we did. We were doing this vital job for a patient who would return in another few weeks and try to hit us, spit on us, and bite us. We'd have to protect ourselves, each other, and him until he got through the violent phase. Laughing together was the way we processed it all.

Lloyd's body would stop seizing in a couple days, then we'd remove the ventilator, take his food orders, and nurture him back to health. He would be downgraded from ICU status to the medical–surgical floor as he gained his independence. He'd then be discharged with the same instructions as always: stop drinking, seek help, stay strong. We all knew this wouldn't be the last time we would see Lloyd or the numerous other patients who frequented our hospital beds. The difference with Lloyd, though, was that we knew he'd be apologetic and ask if he'd hurt anyone. This was a man whose disease was stronger than he was. All we could do was help him each time he showed up on our unit, even if it was relentlessly exhausting. The laughter and distractions kept us all looking at the brighter side of things.

"Nursing is a twenty-four-hour job. There is a reason we work in shifts," Stacy warned as she walked out of Lloyd's room ready to give report to the oncoming shift. As a new grad I was routinely staying late, feeling the need to complete every task I could. The overachiever in me struggled to turn off, ensuring every bit of the day was documented and my patient was taken care of as if they were my own family member. Stacy used this as a teaching moment to show that one can be a good nurse and still delegate to the next shift.

Being a new nurse was thrilling, but it was also draining on me. In addition to the job itself, I would come to know that learning and studying never stopped and we were responsible for advocating not only for our patients but for ourselves as well, something that wasn't a strong suit of mine. Thus, Stacy's warning stayed with me, reminding me to recognize my limits and know when to relinquish responsibility and delegate tasks. I never quite got used to leaving things undone, or to delegating for that matter. Advocating for myself was a lesson I wouldn't learn until much later in my career.

8. Losing Battle
March 2013

We soaked in the last few moments of the unseasonably early spring air before filing in through the glass entrance. A mob of people in white and light blue scrubs herded past the hand-painted mural depicting nurses and nuns caring for patients. We rode in the elevator to our respective floors and clocked in for the start of another day.

"I don't care what happens today, I'm leaving for the ocean tomorrow. We can get through the next twelve hours," Jake said, cheering us on with the hope of having a day that ran smoothly. Jake had started in the ICU the year before I came onboard and was a seasoned nurse in my eyes. The nature of the job and need for comradery drew a group of a dozen of us newer nurses to close friendship, and on this day most of us had the luxury of working together.

Days bright like this one seemed to illuminate the unit—one that was a revolving door of fragile surgical patients, chronic frequent fliers, and people trying to die. On this day sunbeams darted in through patient blinds and filled the nurses' station with rays of cheer. Somehow the sunlight quieted the continuous ringing of alarms and brought an optimistic feel to the morning. This day was most like any other sunny day—until it wasn't.

Jake had the open bed, the coveted and dreaded assignment of having one patient and an empty room, first to admit anyone who might need ICU care. It seemed like fate intercepted his earlier boast by calling a code moments after we'd clocked in.

"Code Blue, fifth floor, room five-two-eight. Attention. Code Blue, fifth floor, room five-two-eight. All teams respond," a calm female voice announced overhead as I heard the code pager vibrate then start chirping at the charge nurse's desk. As if setting off the alarm at a fire station, everyone on the unit jumped into action.

Dread is the initial feeling of knowing there is a life needing saving, especially during our shift report. But the feeling is almost immediately shifted to one of a worker bee mentality in knowing we need to become a team.

Nurses are given a very brief thirty-minute overlap of staff at the beginning and end of each shift to discuss all the details of patient assignments and to have safe handoffs in the hospital. This delicate window of time is often interrupted with phone calls, new admits, and emergencies that can't be planned for and pressure from management to not go into overtime. So, we rushed through reports on patients that could use much more than a mere few moments of discussion about their ailments, hoping we'd covered the highlights and anxious about the coding patient arriving imminently.

Three nurses gathered at the unit's double doors and waited for them to slowly open before quickly jogging toward the elevators, off to get the patient from the telemetry floor. We knew we'd be seeing them in a few short minutes when they brought the dying patient into the ICU where we had all the resources to save a life, so we rushed through the remaining reports on the other patients on the unit. Then we jumped into "go mode," grabbing things we anticipated needing. We instinctively pulled out supplies, turned on the monitor, and laid out cables to be attached to the patient while the respiratory therapist wheeled a ventilator into the room. The completion of each task built excitement in the room for the upcoming adrenaline dump (both for the patient and for us).

The patient arrived and the unit bustled; it was a frenzied scene of scrub-clad bodies moving in different directions. Orders were shouted out while nurses ran to various corners of the unit for medications and other machines needed to help save this patient's life. We desperately tried to correct his critical values as the monitor alarms rang notifying us the unstable patient was teetering at the edge of life. We knew there was family driving in to be with him, and we were trying to buy time until they arrived.

Jake spent the first four hours of his shift in that patient's room doing the job that needed two or more nurses to manage. He was a strong nurse and knew when to ask for help, so we were all glad he was the one handling this situation. We assisted him where we could, jumping in to perform CPR or fetching supplies each time the code button was pressed. Throughout the morning we repeatedly stabilized the patient with chest compressions and Epinephrine, offered last-minute help to Jake, then rushed back to the patients we had all abandoned in the moment. Before noon we had used two code carts to save not only his life but also the life of another coding patient on the unit. We all had our own patients to care for while also keeping an eye on Jake's second patient. Luckily, he was stable and was awaiting a bed on the telemetry unit.

It's mornings like this one that warrant extra staff. The hospital is a fast-paced and unpredictable environment that can require the influx of staff in a moment's notice. Every patient needs medical attention, each a ticking time bomb of physical ailments and emotional needs. If we hadn't stepped in, there would have been no one to help Jake or his other patient all day. It is vital nursing peers run a smooth code together and anticipate one another's needs.

Communicating by instinct creates an unbreakable bond between nursing comrades. Health-care workers experience and handle more traumatic events, usually on a daily basis, than some people ever face in their lifetime. When one faces death and the unexplainable every day and somehow survives situations that incapacitate the average person, it's hard to look at the people in the trenches with you and not trust them with your life.

By late afternoon the family of the dying patient had met the ICU doctor, one of our Sisters, and the ethics committee to discuss end of life. The family, now at the bedside, was ready to sit with their grandpa and let him go. Jake consoled them and answered unanswerable questions about how and why, and a Sister was there to comfort them through their tears.

We were grateful for the decision to bring this man peace, and it released much-needed resources and staff back to the other needs of the unit. We were also thankful that his family was with him while he passed. An oath this Catholic hospital instilled in my baby nursing soul was that *no one dies alone.*

Saving a life isn't an easy task, nor is it guaranteed. Even when everything is done correctly, there are deaths that science can't adequately explain. Maintaining a life that so desperately wants to leave this planet so family members can have their last moments with them is a feat every nurse knows too well.

As nurses, we fight for that life in the bed and the family's right to grieve. We fight with charge nurses who tell us to put the patient in a body bag and prepare for a new admit. There is no grace period to collect yourself or acknowledge the fact you have just crashed from an adrenaline high while you hug the sobbing family members. It is a whirlwind of emotion, and before you have time to finally take that bathroom break, there is a new patient to fill the empty bed. It is relentless, exhausting, and soul-straining. But we live for it.

There is a sixth sense that comes with clinical experience and time. Health-care workers become tuned into sensing when things are about to take a turn for the worse. Nights with full moons always get a little crazier, and we superstitiously never say the word *quiet* out loud for fear of waking some sleeping devil ready to hand us more death, disease, and unexplainable loss.

A good ICU nurse is tuned into the unit as a whole. Not only will they know every detail about their own patients but they also have a good handle on who is on the unit, where the weak nurses are, and who the strong nurses are. They can sense when things begin to go awry. ICUs aren't quiet places. There are too many patients, variables, and monitors for something not to be ringing an alarm at all times.

On first inspection, an onlooker may assume the nurses are running around while ignoring the alarms; however, we know what every alarm is and what it sounds like, and we can probably tell you which patient the alarm belongs to without even looking up. We hear these alarms in our sleep and know them to our core. We anticipate fast heart rates, low oxygen levels, and dropping blood pressures. We know when a respiratory alarm is meaningless, and we certainly know when to get up and run to an event. We also know firsthand that staying tuned into the "meta" of the ICU is exhausting and an additional drain to the physical, emotional, and mental nature of the job.

On this particular morning, after family arrived and we let that dying patient go, we were all on high alert; our senses were extra engaged thanks to the continuous coding of one patient and the knowledge all our patients were critically ill. By the time the afternoon rolled around, we were frazzled and running on fumes. Only a few of us had gotten an actual lunch break, and even if we'd had the chance to consume fuel, we were still run down from the stress of the day.

Losing a patient, while disheartening and tragic, is also sometimes a relief. We were all thankful the nightmare of running a code for six hours had finally ended. It was time to get back to every other patient whose life was fragile. The afternoon looked like it was going to wind down at a good pace, and just in time to get Jake his much-needed break from the overstimulating environment.

Jake's "nothing can bring me down" attitude seemed to linger as he sat to chart. Then, as we all hurried to complete tasks for the day, the mocking sound of the code alarm began to scream from the flashing light above room two—Jake's other patient.

"Code Blue, ICU, room two. Attention. Code Blue, ICU, room two. All teams respond."

Instinctively, everyone ran toward the flashing light, grabbing supplies along the way. Pharmacy hadn't restocked the unit's last code cart yet, so we wheeled it from one bed to the next in preparation for running the same script we had been running all day.

"One, two, three, four . . ." a nurse counted off while starting compressions.

"He's a DNR! Stop compressions!" *Stop compressions?!* This man had just been talking to us a minute ago! The nurse stopped compressions, and we all stood back and watched the monitor as his heart rhythm began to fade.

"Do not resuscitate" the woman repeated loudly, nodding at us with her curly white hair like one of the Golden Girls. A Sister stepped in to verify his code status, then delivered the news of the patient's passing in real time over the phone, remaining on the line to comfort the family. They had already said their goodbyes and would not be coming to see him.

Standing there, stunned and shaken from the day that had unfolded before us, I was unable to come up with a complete thought or words to summarize just one feeling I was cloaked in—shock *and* exhaustion. I also felt sad for the man we had helped and spoken to all day. We'd all cared for him while Jake was saving another life. Every one of us was worn down from fighting for so many patients, and we still had a stack of charting to catch up on. Our shoulders collectively slumped as we fumbled around the room and prepared the patient for the next stage.

Death is a normal part of the job. But despite it being common, it doesn't get any easier. Even a peaceful, anticipated death that has family present, we nurses still feel that loss. We fight for the lives of patients as if they are our own family members. So, both deaths that day felt like defeat. The first one happened after we'd all worked tirelessly together for hours, warding it off with our potions and machines until the family was able to be there. The second one occurred so quickly that it stopped our worlds for a few moments.

Nurses must mourn deaths fairly quickly; there is no room to take it home with us. But we all do. And we are a little snarkier and more jaded about life because of it. Mostly, we hold it in for our rant sessions with fellow nurses, knowing that society at large can't handle the sorrows we consume daily. We have no moment of silence or the chance to cry it out. We swallow our grief and move on with life because we must. There is always another patient who needs us, and our families and communities need us. We must don the brave armor of being totally unscathed from moments that break most people. And we are expected to do it with a smile while catering to the demands that come with working in a health-care system.

9. Deciding to Travel
September 2013

Two years after fate swapped a future in the burn unit for cardiac surgery, I felt I had a pretty good handle on being an intensive care nurse. I wasn't quite ready to take on being in charge, but I itched to grow my medical knowledge and experience. I was confidently handling any admit that came through our cardiac unit, orienting new grads, and building a family of peers who I trusted with my life and were learning to trust me.

Experiencing so many traumatic events with the same people can make you really close. We learned how to read each other in moments of adrenaline dumps and laughed off the insanity of pulling maggots from patient wounds together. We bonded over the cafeteria's infamous Veggie Delight sandwiches while chuckling at horror stories that couldn't be told or even fathomed in different company. It was traumatic, but we were in it together and living our dreams of saving lives.

After two years, I started feeling the unsettled ache of needing to do something more. I was certain healing didn't end with surgery or long-term medications, and I had always been intrigued by natural remedies and the healing touch. I knew the impact massage therapy and physical training could provide and longed to learn more about alternative healing. My peers were seeking certifications and admission into nurse practitioner programs, and I was reaching a plateau. I felt there was so much more that could be brought to the bedside to help our patients heal than what was being offered by Western medicine.

When I first started wanting more from health care, I turned to massage therapy. My friends were beginning master's programs, whereas I wanted to learn more about healing the person as a whole. Western medicine focuses on measurable science in the body and largely disregards the impact the mind and spirit can have in recovery. Even while I attended nursing school I assumed there would be more education on natural remedies and healing alternatives, but the programs are designed to teach the basics and prepare students for the hospital environment. I wanted to know more than what I'd been taught.

Just weeks after securing a spot for a local night program in massage therapy, my friend Emma called for a girls' night. We got dressed up and planned to fill ourselves with our favorite Italian food and catch up. Emma beamed with excitement as she blurted out, "Myles and I are going to travel!" The table erupted with excitement as we fired off questions about location and what they were going to do with their furniture. They were off to travel the country while fulfilling three- to six-month contracts at hospitals in whatever state they landed in.

Driving home that night, it sunk in that two of my closest friends would be leaving, while others would be going off to school. The team was changing. I couldn't ignore the longing in my chest that I, too, had wanted to travel. It was a dream I had put on a shelf while still in school. I laid in bed wide awake that night thinking about the possibility of becoming a travel nurse. After all, I felt pretty confident in the ICU and was itching for something more. Maybe other places performed medicine differently? At three in the morning, I opened my laptop and applied to be a travel nurse, and by the time I woke up, I had a mailbox full of recruiters' messages asking where I wanted to go first. Before I knew it, I withdrew from the massage therapy program and was preparing for life on the road.

10. Finding Arizona
December 2013

I surely wasn't prepared to stay in Evansville, a border town between Indiana and Kentucky. I had only been there three months, and I had seen all I needed to see of the town and the hospital. It was a jarring first assignment that made me question my decision to travel.

The CVICU I was assigned to was small and performed only a couple open-heart surgeries a week. That, and it didn't have the best reputation. The bulk of the patients were there to have sheaths pulled following a visit to the cath lab.

When a patient has a cardiac catheterization, they go to the cardiac catheterization lab, the cath lab, and a metal stent that looks like a coil is used to open up a blocked artery around the heart, much like a viaduct is used to open a waterway. In order to get to the vessel around the heart, a long tube about the diameter of a pencil is inserted (similar to an IV into a blood vessel in the groin), then threaded all the way up to the heart. It truly is a miraculous procedure, and there is nothing like watching someone's symptoms improve and life be saved in mere moments when a cardiologist places a stent and allows blood to flow around the heart again. And all this occurs while the patient is awake and talking!

Following the procedure the patient must lie completely flat for multiple hours after having a nurse hold firm pressure on their groin for at least fifteen minutes to help form a clot. The sheath pull can be a miserable experience for everyone involved, and that is presuming everything goes right. It can be a nightmare, if not fatal, when things go wrong. I had never pulled a sheath in the ICU I had come from, and I suddenly didn't feel ready to be a travel nurse.

My nurse orientater, Paul, guided me through my first removal. Paul was a few years my senior, every bit the nurse I dreamed of becoming, and had been traveling for years by the time our paths crossed. His snarky sense of humor made my stress melt away, and he seemed to know everything. Paul allowed me to ask every ridiculous question a nurse with experience should know but with different monitors, charting system, IV pumps, and no doctor in sight to give orders.

Gulp! The level-one trauma facility I had come from had two doctors on at any given time and a plethora of surgeons who could give direction with a quick call. This facility was different, to say the least. The doctors seemed to end their shift before the night crew even arrived. Complete competency was a must to work there, anticipating what the doctors might order and managing care without a director. *How was I supposed to know what a doctor would order? I'm just a nurse.* Luckily, I had found a travel mentor.

I felt like a student nurse again; I was uncertain whether I was qualified enough to be there, and I was terrified of doing something wrong. After landing in the circus of this hospital, it became very apparent how little I actually knew. But Paul's support helped me continue facing each day and looking at the bright side. He challenged me with hypothetical scenarios and hemodynamic questions, all of which prepared me to be a stronger nurse.

"Arizona?" I questioned my recruiter. "Why would I want to go to the desert? It is probably nothing but tumbleweeds and trailers with snakes hanging from trees."

As I'd continuously run down my bucket list of places I wanted to go, I'd been anxiously anticipating the approval of a Louisiana nursing license to put me close to Mardi Gras. Then my recruiter called and insisted we needed to choose a backup plan because we were running out of time.

Pennsylvania isn't part of the compact license states. This meant each state I wanted to work in required a lengthy application process, excessive fees, and background checks that took anywhere from forty-eight hours to fourteen weeks to complete. Licensing is a hurdle for any traveling nurse, but Arizona's ability to offer a temporary license allowed for short-notice travelers like me to begin working almost immediately. And the fact Paul was heading to Tucson to visit family and take a thirteen-week assignment made my transition to the desert a little easier. I wasn't yet ready to lose my mentor.

As the landscape changed, I became surrounded by mountains and cacti in a terrain foreign to me. It didn't take long to see that Tucson wasn't going to be the rattlesnakes and tumbleweeds of my nightmares after all. Though I could have never imagined I'd plant roots and call it home a decade later, the desert became a resting stop for me to refuel on friendships and sunset hikes before heading out on my next travel nurse adventure.

For the next number of years, I continued to return to the same hospital in Arizona as a nurse traveler. Each visit back to the familiar unit challenged me and helped me grow my skill set. I formed unbreakable bonds with staff members over some of the most intense night shifts that had us admitting sick open-heart patients and responding to catastrophic emergencies. This community hospital had an old-school feel, not only because the nurses themselves were seasoned but also because they maintained an attitude of working cohesively as a team. It felt like my home hospital because of its teamwork mentality and a passion for care. There were high expectations from all staff, and I was surrounded by people who were dedicated to helping others as well as participating in ongoing learning.

11. Traveling Spirit
September 2013 – January 2020

"Wow, you don't travel lightly, do you?" Paul said in his playful, sarcastic tone. I had just finished unpacking our whitewashed second-floor apartment with larger-than-life desert mountain views, and Paul was pointing to the picture frames and table clock I had placed on the rental furniture of our new home away from home.

Home was a *feeling* I had when I was young—it was never a place, and certainly not a place that always felt safe. I knew no matter where I ended up living, I'd be able to call the place *home* if even just for a few weeks. My photos and knickknacks transformed every new casa into a familiar retreat. The instability from my childhood made the transition to travel life relatively easy.

Living my life in three-month increments was both exhilarating and exhausting. By my second assignment, I realized which items were worth traveling with and which I could forgo in exchange for more cargo space. Along with my collection of clothes and shoes, I made sure to bring some key kitchen items: a good knife, my favorite mixing/straining bowl combo, a coffee pot, and a Crock-Pot. I enjoyed baking and found meal prepping easiest with weekly Crock-Pot meals. I also always had my fishing poles with me, a Tupperware full of lotions, potions, and hair accessories, and more baskets filled with picture frames and home decor trinkets. For companionship, I maintained a stream of beta fish in a small portable fishbowl that rode shotgun to each new destination.

I purchased trash cans and hangers more times than I can count, as I never had the space to repack these items. I traded a broom and vacuum for a no-shoes approach and found out a container of bleach wipes can clean up just about anything. By the time things needed a deep clean, my contract would be up and I'd be on the move again, grateful for the cleaning deposit I'd paid when moving in.

I loved everything about traveling, from relying on GPS to forgetting which apartment number I lived in. I looked forward to the adventure of finding my "new" grocery store and thinking about which route I would take to and from work. I enjoyed learning about various hospital layouts, new ways of caring for patients, and the machines I had never seen before.

Though it was easier to have my travel company find an apartment for me in each location, I learned I could save money by finding my own place. Whether I was settling into a cozy one-room cabin for the winter or watching hot-air balloons ascend in Napa, I adored burrowing in, finding a perch for my Penguins hockey gnome, and unpacking my clothes into new dressers for new adventures in new towns with new people.

I spent my off time exploring my new surroundings. Being alone thrilled me; I could go and see whatever I wanted. Traveling 2,500 miles away from home made a six-hour drive to visit a national park seem like a weekend getaway rather than a daunting trek. Travel nursing inspired me to make the most of my free time and offered experiences I could have never dreamed of as a little girl.

Three months was all it took for me to decide whether I liked a hospital or not. The first few weeks were usually spent in a fog of apologies as I wandered the halls, learning my way around and asking for help. Charting would always take me a bit longer as I learned the new system.

At the four- to six-week mark, I knew which doctors I preferred and what staff members I could most trust. It's about this time that I'd hand out my door code cheat sheet to the newest travelers on the unit. Nearing the nine-week mark I'd have proven myself as competent and gained the trust of the team. By that time, I would have made a handful of friends and could finally find all the supplies, just in time for my recruiter to call and ask where I wanted to go next.

Inside the walls of each hospital, I acquired tools, learned about new medications, and repeated familiar techniques. I got to see firsthand how demographics and socioeconomics affect health, and I learned about new cultures. I witnessed families celebrate life and mourn the loss of their child. I sat with people of all faiths and listened to patients who felt hopeless and weary. I fumbled through language barriers, cared for the victim and the criminal, and watched as Natives smudged the room of a dying elder. I witnessed the strength love and community can have on healing and saw what neglect of the sick can lead to. This world is a beautiful and tragic place, and I got a front-row seat to humanity through travel nursing.

12. Atheist in a Foxhole
February 2011

I thrived under the pressure of being a cardiac intensive care nurse. The fragility of life hanging on the balance and having a hand in saving it fueled the passion I had for my own life. Every day was a challenge, and while the job eventually became more predictable, it was never easy. Patients seemed to get more complex, and serious procedures became more common.

Nurses are translators of medical jargon for patients and their family members. We need to understand something at a level that we can deliver news and answer all the questions that may arise. We must be able to deliver information in a way the recipient can understand, allow them time to process it, then return to answer questions. We are often the bridge between patients and how they understand their own health. We need time, energy, and patience—three crucial factors in communicating, and three things the current health-care system no longer allows for.

Healing involves much more than the salt water we hang in your IV bag or the opium derivative we give to you to swallow the pain away or the dressing we change every six hours to avoid infection. Healing requires space to accept that our bodies are unable to keep up in that moment. It requires us to step back and see what could have been done differently to avoid this outcome, to remove or improve what made us sick or caused the injury, then to take the time, energy, and patience to implement those changes. In acute care and emergency medicine, the recovery time following an injury has become nonexistent. We rush patients out of the hospital to go home alone or with family members who have no medical knowledge and potentially no compassion for this human who needs it.

In American society today the ill seem to be discarded. Families send relatives to hospitals to get better and sometimes we make them worse or add a new illness, new medication, or new confusing statistics. Everything is rushed, standardized, and deemed not important until one is literally fighting for their life. Then they get the attention they deserve. When your heart loses its will to keep going, we jump on your chest, determined to live for you. We push through your cracking ribs with locked elbows and stacked hands while counting the beats to the Bee Gees' song "Staying Alive"—an ironic and necessary tune with exactly the number of beats per minute we need to hopefully restart your heart. Meanwhile, another nurse injects a toxic chemical into your system with the hope your cells will come back to life and fight again. While our brains calculate oxygen levels, we anticipate the needs of the doctors filing in and out, ready to run through the most recent lab values and push more Epinephrine. Our brains and our hearts go into lifesaving mode for you.

Soldiers often say there are no atheists in foxholes, and I'd say it applies to any situation where someone is fighting to save another's life. Our own hearts beat harder and faster to revive yours while also looking up to whatever power is out there, to whatever power is more definitive than science, and we pray to it for help.

However, our prayers aren't always to help save this life. Sometimes we pray the family sees the pain they are putting their family member through, or the patient no longer has to suffer on the brink of death anymore. Sometimes we pray that no one else starts to die that day because when one code alarms, there are bound to be others. We pray our little hearts out while multitasking critical chores.

If the life is saved, we try to neutralize the situation. While the body in the bed may be clinically alive with a heartbeat on the monitor, we know this is just the beginning of a long road ahead—a long journey of their body trying to live for itself and of their soul being saved through it all. We hope they wake up and return to life as they knew it, but there is no way to tell. So, we answer the questions the best we know how.

"He's stable. Now we wait," we say, referring to the omnipresent God factor we're not allowed to utter in the name of science.

The number of times my mouth has uttered these words is countless. Science stands proudly in opposition to belief in a higher power, but truth be told, when you're on the inside of it and you have the most capable scientists by the bedside and the ideal patient and all the right circumstances occur, there are matters out of our control. We can't help but shrug our shoulders and admit we don't know. While this is the unspoken truth underlying all of medicine, we spend very little time investigating or believing in that supernatural power. We barely acknowledge it at all except to tell families we have no idea what the outcome will be.

And when we aren't able to save the life in the bed, everyone's energy shifts. The room quiets, though never really stopping in motion, and we wait for the doctor to call it.

"Time of death: thirteen twenty-seven."

Our heads hang and we admit defeat, and for the slightest moment, time seems to linger. Then the familiar sound of gloves being pulled off solidifies another life lost. Staff begin to clean up the garbage and syringes thrown about the room as evidence of the emergency. We cover the bruised and lifeless body with a blanket and try to hide the bloodstains on the bed with clean linens. We replace the pillow taken from under their head during intubation and wipe the dried blood from their face. We lower the bed and, out of habit, raise the side rails. We pull chairs from other rooms and place them alongside the bedside and place a brand-new box of tissues close by.

For me, it's time to don a new hat. I must be with the family members, whom I don't know. I need to look them in the eyes and honestly say that we did everything we could. I must put aside my to-do list for my other patients to honor the life lost, if only for a few minutes. I listen to them tell stories of their loved one and offer a shoulder to cry on.

So many times I want them to know I loved the patient too. Even if I only knew the ill version of them for a few hours, I cared for them as if they were my own blood. I worked for them, I fought for them, I prayed for them. But I don't. I allow the family to grieve and help soak up any of the pain I can.

13. HS—Hour of Sleep
February 2011 – August 2020

Contrary to belief, patients don't stop being sick when the sun goes down. Emergencies relentlessly unfold while the ill continue to require twenty-four-hour care. Due to the perceived downtime the night shift has, more tasks are added to the nocturnal ("noc") shift duties, including bathing, dressing, and IV tube changing, as well as general unit maintenance on top of regular patient care and documentation.

Fighting to maintain knowledge and judgment on a night shift when the only thing your body wants to do is sleep can be a difficult struggle for hospital staff. Lack of sleep inhibits critical thinking skills, skills vitally needed because most medical teams are home asleep in their beds. There is an added level of competency a night shift requires, and it made me want to be a stronger nurse.

There are definite perks to working daytime hours. Having doctors and resources readily available, eating regular meals, seeing the sunshine, and feeling well rested are some of my personal favorites. While the hospital doesn't shut down at night, there is a significant slowdown in mayhem that allows for the smallest amount of extra time for decision-making and care. For me, it was during the hours of 7:00 p.m. to 7:30 a.m. when I felt I could serve my patients best, regardless of the toll it was taking on my life. I took day-shift contracts sporadically when they were available, if for no other reason than to feel human for three months. The stress of the day shift never changed, but with adequate sleep and a more human routine, it was manageable.

Moving every three to six months while learning new hospital systems was a lot in and of itself. So, working nights meant less administration and testing, fewer families to inform and console, and more time to actually care for the patients. I preferred the less busy environment the night shift offered.

A significant requirement of the job is working nights, weekends, and holidays. Having a job in health care requires sacrifice, and it is not for the faint of heart. As a young twenty-something whose biggest goal was to find adventure on my days off, the unpredictable schedule fit my flexible life. Those of us who weren't starting families survived on a rotating schedule and the few extra pennies working the undesirable hours brought, although the shift differential never accumulated enough to make up for the lost years the lack of sleep took (and will continue to take) from our lives.

Staff working the night and weekend shifts were granted a bonus of pennies on the dollar for staying awake against their circadian rhythm. We were trained to use our gifts—our hearts and passions—for good and to sell our souls for the almighty dollar. It was a small bonus for willingly avoiding the dreaded rounding of administration, untimely testing, and relentless family interruptions. We had altered mealtimes, and we delayed tasks like grocery shopping and running errands. I didn't mind avoiding crowds during peak hours, and with enough coffee, I could pull all-nighters. The "shift diff" was to accommodate for any semblance of a "normal" life we gave up to care for others.

Now, I never thought nurses made a lot of money, but I saw them earn enough to raise families. Nursing had appeal for me because it has flexible hours, a world of different avenues to travel down, and job security. As long as there are humans, nurses are needed. But "rich nurse" never had that call. The job is physically, mentally, and emotionally draining, but the wage seemed fair enough for the work I endured. Besides, I wanted to be there. I wanted to touch the lives of those who were broken, to bring them a warm blanket and soft smile in their dark times, and to manage drip titrations like I knew what I was doing.

Working the night shift often felt like being on an unmanned ship with nothing but a skeleton crew of people and orders. Anyone who wasn't absolutely necessary for keeping humans alive went home. The rest of us walked empty stairwells and dark hallways to vending machines, bouncing between trying to keep the peace and responding to emergencies.

On the rare occasion the shift was *quiet,* a forbidden word inside the walls of any hospital, we did activities to keep our minds engaged. We had to stay ready to respond to sudden alarms or changes but also be careful not to upset the delicate balance of peaceful patients. So, we reviewed charts, studied disease processes, chugged coffee, and told medical horror stories to get to know each other the way night-shifters do. Then, after hours of being awake against our circadian rhythm, we needed to safely drive home, sleep while the sun was up, and prepare to do it all over again. Our bodies somehow survived the abuse we demanded of them.

14. Toxic Relationship
February 2011 – Current Day

I used to joke about going to work to socialize, but I genuinely thrived when going into the hospital. Being surrounded by intelligent, compassionate, capable people who love life and humans—what is more fulfilling than that? I went to work happy and excited every day because I was happy and hopeful. I found the field compelling and every moment fulfilling—it filled my soul to the brim! Until it didn't anymore.

Falling in love with ICU wasn't too difficult at first. I adjusted well to the shining lights, demanding hours, and myriad of bizarre experiences I'd had during the first twenty-odd years of life. I was getting to comfort the sick and save lives, all while getting paid for it. The frequent rush of adrenaline and the unspoken understanding we were all in this field together felt like having a never-ending family everywhere I went. But my love affair with nursing was losing its allure just as quickly as the ongoing withdrawal of our resources.

Hospital nursing staff typically work three twelve-and-a-half-hour shifts in a week. The thirty-six hours is considered full time, and it's not uncommon to hit the forty-hour mark as one shift bleeds into the next, as our environment is wildly unpredictable.

Working three days a week seems appealing until the days are chopped up throughout the week and you're on a schedule of working every other day and weekends with no set routine. There is no structure in our scheduling, much to our dismay.

Picking up overtime hours is a luxury in our field and can piece together the choppy schedule. Overtime opportunities are abundant as patients continuously flow through hospital corridors and staffing needs grow. For us, management solicited overtime shifts daily via text, tugging on our heartstrings and asking us to give up our self-care time for our patients and our peers. Our forty-hour weeks turn into fifty or sixty hours in our effort to show up for those who need us.

Early on in my career, units were staffed well enough that we could take an actual break away from patient care while the charge nurse and other staff answered call bells and untimely emergencies. When I worked in California, for example, resource nurses were staffed without patients so they could relieve nurses from their duties to ensure breaks. Nurses enjoyed picking up this extra shift as it was a way to help their peers without committing to the responsibility of a full shift assignment. It was a welcome break for both the resource nurse and staff nurse who needed an escape from the ringing bells and attention to detail required at the bedside.

No matter the shift, day or night, breaks help to reset the mind and give us a moment to gather our thoughts and put fuel in our bodies so we can maintain the clarity and stamina it takes to survive this calling. But as the years crept forward, break times were becoming a thing of the past.

While the keepers of time had no problem docking us for thirty minutes of unpaid lunch, the facility itself seemed to forget to give us adequate time to take an actual break. We inhaled many meals while talking on the phone with the lab or after rushing into the bathroom to pee for the first time in ten hours. Regardless of the fact many of us learned to eat on the run didn't make us any less worthy of getting breaks. As hospital staffing began becoming more scarce, so did the opportunity for having time away to regroup and refresh. Charge nurses had assignments of their own, and soon there were no extra staff available to cover for anyone.

These changes were happening at each new placement I had. Management remained unfazed when I expressed safety concerns for missed break times or unsafe float assignments. My choice was to fall in line or they'd cancel my contracts. I did not have the opportunity to advocate for myself and set limits if I wanted to keep my job.

In retrospect, perhaps I should have walked out, but my heart broke for the patients lying in their beds. I was sure the care I was going to struggle through providing over the next twelve hours would be better than what the other nurses could offer after having to absorb extra patients because I walked off the unit.

I longed to know how nurses with twenty- and thirty-years' experience continued to show up to what was beginning to feel like a nightmare rather than a calling. My friends and I sarcastically referred to our jobs as "toxic boyfriends," and we practiced telling off management for mistreating us. But we continued to show up despite the abuse to support our patients and peers. There was dark humor in us laughing off the field's obvious shortcomings as we teased about finding new careers and poked fun at the toxic environment we were tolerating in the name of patient care.

As a traveler, I was first to float and first to be called in. Travelers are utilized in any capacity the hospital's matrix might need. Floating to units out of my wheelhouse of specialty, with more patients, fewer resources, and no idea where supplies were made each float shift exponentially more difficult.

I don't know of any other jobs that throw employees into a new specialty in a moment's notice, without training, while still expecting the management of the well-being and safety of patient lives. Without so much as a "thanks for the help," float staff are sent to various units that have staff and doctors they've never met. They become responsible for the care and advocacy of patients with diseases they're not familiar with and unit routines they don't know. Additionally, they are given discharge instructions they've never read before and must educate patients on procedures they really don't fully understand themselves.

I had experience in ICU, but it didn't mean I knew how to do every nursing role in the hospital. That didn't matter, however; a warm body is a warm body when money and lives are at stake. I struggled to keep up with six to eight patients, not knowing how to turn off the critical-care nurse in myself. I longed to have the skills of the floor nurses who managed to handle every hiccup with ease, and I wanted to take care of many more patients than I was able to. It was a safety concern for the patients and me.

Because patients are rarely sent home directly from the ICU, I had to learn about discharging on my own. As a new traveler, I approached the process the way I wanted discharge instructions explained to me. I pulled up a seat, pen in one hand, highlighter in the other. Page by page, I sat with my patients to review each section, answer questions, and give them time to learn the information. Sure, the extra twenty minutes were moments I didn't have in my schedule to give up, even after I was pulled aside by management on multiple occasions and told to speed up my discharges. But I wasn't there to turn beds for a profit, I was there for the patient.

The intimate time I spent answering questions about discharge with my patients revealed to me how little the general population under-stood things I presumed they knew. Most patients were surprised to find out acetaminophen and Tylenol are the same thing and ibuprofen and Tylenol are *not*. I saw firsthand it is a privilege to have common knowledge of health concerns and how the human body works. A large role of nursing is educating patients about medications, something that should accompany every pill pass. In an ideal world the eager nurse in me was giddy and ready to educate people on the risks and benefits of medications, but there was barely enough time to complete my numerous tasks as it was.

The familiar hospital I'd traveled back to in the desert suddenly no longer had a position for me. Night shifts were taking a toll on me, and I was aching for a break from patient care; I no longer felt like I was able to make a difference. I had a friend who had left the bedside to be a liaison for a rehabilitation hospital, and she raved about the position. It had daylight hours, a set schedule, and a cute dress code! So, I decided to break up with the bedside.

The Monday-to-Friday job allowed me to have a weekly routine that included regular workouts and time for food prepping. My circadian rhythm began to realign, and I was grateful for the change of scenery, though the autonomy of this new role and working out of my truck were a huge adjustment from the confines of a hospital. I was pleased the position still allowed me to interact with patients when I evaluated them for admittance to an acute rehab program, but although I believed in the hospital and the profound effects acute rehab could offer, I still didn't feel like I was making a difference. The requirements for eligibility for admittance were specific, and even if we did find a candidate who checked all the boxes, we then had to fight insurance companies for justification. I was continually perplexed as to why insurance companies would refuse care to patients who needed it most, and I soon became irate with a system that didn't seem to prioritize the people it claimed to serve.

It was an uphill battle, and I wasn't given the opportunity to follow up with the patients I had placed. The feeling of not being able to help enough people or in ways they needed was emotionally overwhelming for me. We did earn a bonus when we reached admission goals, but the money didn't make up for all the people I couldn't help.

I visited doctors' offices in between admitting patients, booking lunches to teach about inpatient rehab while battling other reps in the offices' already full lunch schedule. The office staff complained about restaurant choices and barely paid attention to the information accompanying the free meal. Doctors skirted out of the office, careful to avoid the ever-hounding reps. I was bitter about the ungratefulness, scoffing at the thought of even getting a lunch break. I often thought about the nurses who worked long past their thirteen-hour shifts inside the hospitals and never got to eat.

Before long, my heart ached to be back at the bedside where every shift provided the chance to make an impact on someone's life, but the urgency of intensive care and the revolving door made it feel like I was physically doing more work, so I somehow convinced myself I was making a difference. My goal had been to stay out of the hospital for a year, but I returned to the night shift within eight months and continued to travel. The bedside and I were getting back together.

15. Breaking Down
April 2019

It was becoming apparent that the same issues were occurring at hospitals all across the US. Budget cuts were removing clerical staff and increasing nurse-to-patient ratios. Nurses were becoming laden with more than just the care of patients. Suddenly, answering phones, entering orders, transporting patients, and even basic janitorial tasks were added to the already full plate of the bedside staff. There were fewer hands to care for the patients, while the patients' acuity and needs increased. To add to any good staffing cut was the addition of more audits and checklists to ensure all new tasks were being accomplished.

Routine inspections loomed at every hospital, with State visits to ensure we were doing things by the book, even when there was a staffing shortage. The added pressure was palpable among staff who were already stretched thin. Nurse-to-patient ratios had been a hot-button topic since I had first become a nurse and were constantly being threatened no matter where I was placed.

Each nurse is assigned a set number of patients to take responsibility for during their shift. Depending on the type of unit a nurse works on and the acuity of the patients in their care, a safe nurse-to-patient ratio is decided. When working in an intensive care unit with a patient on life support and requiring minute-by-minute monitoring, a nurse *should* have just two patients at most. A nurse on a unit with patients who have no monitoring needs and can walk themselves to the bathroom might have five to eight patients in their care, for example.

Safe staffing ratios have been a long-term concern for nurses because they are regularly forced to take on more responsibilities with fewer resources. Nursing licenses were becoming compromised by people not at the bedsides making the in-the-moment lifesaving decisions required of a nurse. Nevertheless, nurses were being pushed to take on more patients than reasonably safe to care for, as if they didn't already have too many tasks.

My time as a traveler felt like a double-edged sword. On one hand, I could leave hospitals if the working conditions felt unsafe or unmanageable. The luxury of detaching and moving on always prepared me to claim being a travel nurse as my defense for not willing to cover up for a hospital that didn't actually employ me. On the other hand, however, it became apparent these issues weren't localized and quality care was becoming more difficult to provide in most health-care facilities.

The tolerance for abuse among staff was wearing thin. We rumbled among ourselves, disgruntled with the system and irritated that the world assumed we simply played with doctors' stethoscopes and had time to play cards.

16. Called to the Frontlines
March 2020 – April 2020

I've always been a bit reckless by nature. I impulsively have a habit of acting first and then dealing with hiccups as they come. It's not that I don't care about or consider consequences, it is my innate wild nature and surviving a childhood I never should have that made me fearless toward life's challenges. I lived for the thrill of simply being alive, and like my other nursing peers, I had an air of "not me" when it came to catching the COVID-19 virus. So I responded with an automatic yes when the request came to serve humans at a time when the rest of the world was instructed to isolate.

For the first time in my life I had a place to call home. I was surrounded by the most beautiful healing mountains and in a location that allowed me to spend ample time outdoors, something I loved doing. Unfortunately, God had other reasons for settling me in the desert—to survive the biggest fall of my life and heal my broken soul that only wanted one thing: to take care of others.

At the very beginning of the outbreak, hospital staff proactively wore masks we were then instructed to remove. My brain couldn't comprehend this order when we were potentially facing a respiratory virus. Reluctantly, we removed them at the threat of being sent home for ensuing panic in our patients. A mere twenty-four hours later, State guidelines mandated every health-care worker wear *two* masks to protect themselves against the deadly virus we were facing.

The first few weeks of COVID had everyone on edge, ready to run a code and save lives, all while ignoring the fear in our souls. We understood illness and its transmission. We were used to standing next to death on a daily basis, so COVID wasn't a totally different experience for us other than sensing the fear ravaging society and leaking into the halls of the hospital. We tried to ignore it, show up to work, and not fret about catching it in the same way we didn't spend much time fretting about catching other viruses, such as MRSA or VRE. At the time it was still early in the process of things; we only had a handful of COVID patients in our small hospital, but it felt manageable. The drama being displayed on the news hadn't hit Arizona, yet. I did have family I hadn't heard from in a while and long-lost friends reach out to see how I was doing or to get an inside scoop from a nurse in the middle of it. I didn't really have any more knowledge than they had, and I remained chipper and hopeful for a cure. We were going to conquer this virus, and everything would be back to normal before long.

I wasn't frightened about going to work, I just felt moderately filthier than I did on a normal day and was annoyed the new mask mandate was causing my face to form acne. My drives to and from the hospital were peaceful; I enjoyed the empty roads and beautiful views. Life was eerily calm, and I liked it. I was happy to be in my new permanent home where I could look up at my forever mountains while I used my skills to help save lives during this pandemic. *I had purpose.*

Prior to the COVID outbreak, it wasn't uncommon to have patients in isolation for MRSA or C. diff. COVID wasn't the first wave of a virus that required isolation and seclusion, but it was the biggest in a long time. We spent our pre-shift huddles reviewing skin-care protocols and safe techniques for repositioning our paralyzed and sedated patients.

Due to the severity of coughing COVID patients had while intubated, they needed to be completely paralyzed. Because these patients lacked the ability to communicate or move, it became the nurses' responsibility to rotate them onto their bellies during every shift in an effort to promote lung involvement and circulation and provide pressure relief. So, we gowned up every day and went room to room turning patients of all sizes and shapes, carefully managing the multiple medications infusing through IV lines and the ventilator breathing for them. Feeding tubes and Foley catheters were also carefully rotated along with the patient.

It took at least four people to complete a safe patient rotation and anywhere from twelve to forty-five minutes per patient depending on their status. At 9:00 every morning the "turn team," as we charmingly nicknamed the nurses, stepped away from their own patients to make sure all thirty-plus adult patients were prone for the day.

Each day we received an update on how many new cases were reported in our area. "Skeleton crew" took on a whole new meaning. If you weren't the nurse giving direct patient care or a doctor there to see one of the patients, then you were not permitted on the unit. No exceptions. No dietary, case management, or pharmacy tech. Lab techs were allowed in sparingly, and of course x-ray had to come in, but other than that, the unit was a lonely island: it was just us and our intubated, sedated, paralyzed, proned, dying patients.

While caring for my patients I also took pride in educating the handful of new grads and telling forgotten war stories of H1N1. A decade earlier the US had been struck with an H1N1 pandemic that left many innocent and otherwise healthy people struggling for life. I was brand new to nursing, and our ICU slowed down to allow care for the patients in beds that looked like spaceships rotating around paralyzed bodies. Like a ride at a carnival, these beds locked patients in and mechanically turned them onto their stomachs, allowing for greater surface area of the lungs to attempt oxygenation. Each spaceship patient had their own nurse, someone to monitor the many various wires and tubes needed to maintain their delicate life.

Now, during COVID, I couldn't help but draw comparisons; I had been down this road before. This time, however, we didn't have fancy spaceship beds, and staffing rarely allowed for just one nurse to be focused on one critically ill patient at a time.

By April 2020 it had become absurd and reckless to talk to anyone in the same room without a mask on. I was lonely. Devastatingly lonely. Staff took turns eating lunch in solitude in the break room with masks off to keep "cross contamination" to a minimum. Every door to a patient room was closed, which made the unit eerily quiet. IV poles lined the hall marking every new room and representing a patient who was locked inside the glass corridor fighting off the virus. Trails of orange extension cords ran along the hallways providing the much-needed outlets for the additional equipment outside patient room doors. Equipment that at any other time would have been deemed a safety and privacy risk if placed in the hall had become the norm.

Like a first-grade project, paper bags with names of nurses written on them were taped to doors to hold our precious masks, masks loaded with staples hanging on frayed straps to be used for as many days as we could get them to last. Our gowns and other personal protective equipment (PPE) hung by suction cups in yellow bags. We were required to don this gear every time we entered a patient room.

Muffled ventilator alarms rang periodically from the other side of closed doors, reminding us there were people lying inside these fish-bowls. Ninety percent of the patients were intubated and unable to interact, so exhausted staff were kept busy changing infusion bags and performing other tasks that basic ICU care required.

Symptoms were difficult to manage early on, and a lot of time was spent comforting people we had no answers for, silently panicking, and trying to avoid the near inevitable intubation. There hadn't been enough staff pre-COVID, and now every bed in the hospital was taken. Beds were placed in hallways and corridors, places never intended for patient care, with only a few nurses available to them. It was wartime—controlled chaos that at any moment could burn down the hospital. We did our best to keep everything as calm as possible for our patients, their families, and each other. We knew it was stressful times, though we somehow managed. We were fueled off the adrenaline rush of saving lives and a new and lowered threshold of disregard for our own lives.

From a nurse's perspective, a patient's family members can either radically help in healing or terribly interfere with care. Truth be told, the isolated units during the early stages of COVID were a relief. Not having family members to contend with gave us a break from more people needing more things from us.

No matter the intention, when someone is visiting a friend or family member in the hospital and wants to make even light conversation with the nursing staff, they are requiring a nurse's attention, attention that could be given to a patient or to self-care for a quick swig of water or run to the restroom. So, not having additional people in the unit certainly lightened our workload—at first.

At the beginning of the pandemic, it was as if families were too scared to call in. The entire world was in a state of shock and awe, no one had any answers, and it seemed like society knew those on the inside of health care didn't have answers either. Calls were short, and people respected we were busy, something that gave us back some of the time and energy we needed to care for the masses of people dying.

We intubated, sedated, dropped feeding tubes, and held onto hope for helpless bodies in hopeless situations. We knew if someone got to the point where they needed a breathing tube, it was likely they would die with it in. We didn't tell this to our patients, of course, but we tried our very best to wait until the last moment to take their freedom. We put on a smile under our masks, called their families, and spoke calming words softly in the patients' ears. It would all be okay, we said, trying to believe it ourselves. Meanwhile, the rest of the team buzzed around preparing the room for intubation like out of a scene in the movie *ET*.

It wasn't long into the pandemic when hospitals began implementing the use of iPads for video calls with family members. When someone's health began taking a turn for the worse and putting them on life support became imminent, the staff would grab an iPad and call family members so the patient had the chance to say goodbye. The pandemic changed the way we saw things. We realized once patients were put on the ventilator they were unlikely to come off it, so we helped them cherish the last few breaths they had by making those calls before they had to rely on machines to live for them with no cure in sight. We knew those last moments of having energy to breathe and talk were likely their last even though we'd still be turning and caring for their bodies months later.

On the other side of death was the pride we felt in showing up when no one else could. We had pride for being the ones who "saved the day," comforted the sick, and sat with the dying, tasks that made me want to become a nurse in the first place. We rallied together and jumped in as a team. No one complained, and although we were all terrified, we were all ready to stand in the face of doom while subtly ignoring the fact we were risking our own lives as well as those of our loved ones at home. It wasn't the pandemic that brought out these characteristics in us, however; the pandemic just put a microscope on what we were already doing.

Early on in my nursing career before I became a traveling nurse, my home hospital was up for our annual State inspection. During the visit, one of our patients coded and the team rushed in to provide CPR, crack the crash cart, feel for a pulse, administer lifesaving medications, and console the family. Success! We'd saved another life, and this particular code had run incredibly smoothly from start to finish. There'd been closed-loop communication and clear roles, allowing us to save the life in minutes.

In the debrief later that afternoon, our spiky-haired manager grinned half-heartedly while reviewing the State's report: "I have good news and I have bad news. We were commended on our teamwork, and you were praised for your knowledge and timeliness. However, we were penalized for rushing to the care of the patient before putting on the required gowns and masks for this MRSA isolation patient." We all groaned and began to argue.

"It's MRSA," the bedside nurse said as we rolled our eyes and huffed. The virus was in the patient's urine and the patient had a Foley catheter, making it contained and unlikely for us to catch and transfer. But this fact didn't matter; the life saved was overshadowed by a slap on the wrist for not obeying isolation precautions. There was no emphasis on the fact we were risking our own lives and health; instead, the report highlighted our insubordination.

Fast-forward nine years and the hospital where I was working didn't have the appropriate PPE and was informing us, in so many words, that our lives were not valued. But we continued dancing along as PPE requirements changed by the shift, then by the hour. We were constantly changing the types of masks we wore and accommodating the rules for how many days used PPE was "effective," all while simplifying patient care amid a crisis of supplies and help. As for gloves, in times of famine we were told not to double glove after demanding the week before to double glove for fear of contamination. Our supplies were used long past the one-and-done instructions drilled into our brains previously. The rules no longer seemed to matter; our only goal for a large chunk of the pandemic was to keep patients alive.

17. Walmart Hero
April 2020

Things seemed to flow on as best they could, and we were falling into a familiar routine. Our spirits were waning, but we remained hopeful. Comradery was abundant and community support poured in, something I'll always remember about that time. The community really came together to love and support us. It felt a little like over-kill; we were doing what we always did, just with more PPE on. The abundance of gifts of food and encouragement felt unwarranted. So many people were supporting us for putting our lives on the line, but we had done that every day throughout our careers.

Meal after meal arrived from local organizations in gratitude for us taking care of their community. Handwritten cards from kids calling us heroes lined the walls of the hospital's entrance, and donations of hand-sewn masks and food were delivered daily. All this love kept us going.

Food is a love language and one that nurses accept graciously. Payment and gifts from patients aren't expected, but it's always a surprise to receive treats with accompanying cards sharing thanks for the care we gave to them or their loved ones. These notes hang proudly on every bulletin board, in every breakroom, and in every hospital I've ever worked in. Knowing our care makes a difference reminds us we are valued and inspires us to keep fighting for our patients.

My friends and I didn't particularly like being called heroes. Our actions were not heroic; we were caring for people like we always had: giving them medications; coaching them on breathing techniques; reminding them to drink enough water and make healthy food choices; educating the same patient we'd discharged the week prior, the month prior, and the year prior with the same discharge instructions: "Take care of yourself"—which for nurses, was something easier said than done.

Early in the pandemic before restrictions were made, before the hospitals knew what to do, and when everyone was panic-shopping and leaving barren toilet paper shelves, I had been at Walmart picking up some provisions for a potluck at work that evening. When you work a thirteen- or even fourteen-hour shift, you have little time to make an additional trip to the grocery store between feeding yourself and your family and finding time to sleep. Running to the store in my scrubs was just part of the job. I basically lived in scrubs.

I braced myself for backlash. I was ready to get scolded for having my (unbeknownst to anyone else—CLEAN) scrubs on and carrying the virus (this is not scientifically sound) because of videos showing nurses being insulted for wearing their uniforms in public. While I was walking down the pasta aisle, I passed an elderly gentleman in an old, loose-fitting baseball jacket. The navy blue had faded to white around the cuffs and elbows. His smile was even older and kinder.

"Hey . . . " he said with a quiver, pausing to gather the attention of the many other pasta aisle shoppers. He stood with one arm outstretched toward me and a finger trembling in my direction. I was leery of what might come out of his mouth as he drew onlookers. The quiver made me think he wasn't used to being the center of attention, but the hesitation and shakiness in his soft voice caused everyone around the carb-lovers aisle to take notice. A toothy grin crept across his face, and I braced myself.

"Isn't that what superheroes wear?" he said with a lighthearted chuckle.

Bystanders looked at me. I flushed and had no idea what to say.

"I . . . I . . . I'm just doing what I was put here to do," I choked out after releasing the breath I'd been holding in fear of being attacked. I smiled bashfully and refused to give in to the urge I had to hug this stranger with all my might. I still didn't feel like a hero.

Today, I love reflecting on the beautiful feelings I had of watching the world come together to stand behind our health-care workers during such a dark time. Yes, we needed support and encouragement, but it was the compassion for the neighbor or friend who might be lying in a hospital bed that was kept alive with this support. It was as if the whole world paused and allowed time and space for the healing of the sick.

18. Silver Lining
May 2020 – December 2020

On May 14, 2020, our local Air Force base planned to honor first responders and frontline workers with a flyover. I was scheduled to be off that day and was anticipating the event with excitement. I loved it when the Air Force performed maneuvers over our city. I was like a little kid waiting for fireworks to start as I stood staring up at the cloudless sky.

Receiving a salute from the military was the most honorable act in my mind aside from New York and other areas clapping and banging pots and pans at 7:00 p.m. daily for a number of weeks. I didn't crave accolades, but the appreciation reminded me that what we were doing was meaningful to someone somewhere.

I could feel the rumble of jet engines in my stomach as a knot gathered in my throat. I waited motionless with my head cocked back, parallel to the sky, anxious to catch sight of the planes as they soared overhead. Flying in a V formation, three metallic angels cut through the sea of blue, turning the rumble into a roar. I shivered and felt unworthy. Awestruck with gratitude, I thought about how many people it might take to coordinate a flyover. The love felt too much to bear.

Without taking my eyes off them, I followed their soaring path over the backyard and to the driveway where I stood watching them in awe as they continued toward the city limits. I couldn't breathe. *This was for me. This was for us. This was for all the hell and turmoil we were going through.* I was amazed anyone wanted to honor us to this extent, and the flyover was enough to reenergize me and keep my heart focused on our patients. Going to work became a little easier for the next few weeks.

The community support was keeping me alive as neighborhoods and cities continued cheering for us. There were nursing discounts for shoes and services and even free food for us tired "heroes." I still wasn't used to the title and didn't feel right taking advantage of the gifts after being trained by hospitals to not accept presents from patients. My tone changed, however, when a local law firm offered to complete free wills for frontline workers. I jumped at the opportunity to save thousands on the legal document. Having the new financial responsibility of a home and beginning to realize I was actually putting my own life on the line encouraged me to take advantage of this opportunity.

Over the years I had advised many patients and families to ensure they had living wills in place long before the need for one arose. Not everyone wants to live indefinitely with the help of machines and be reliant on others to turn, bathe, and care for them.

In medicine, we presume everyone wants to live despite long-lasting disabilities and impairments, but many people wish to have their dignity and peace remain intact when the moment arises. And the moment will arise for all of us eventually.

The stark reality of death being absolute rather than unimaginable emphasized a "quality over quantity" approach to life and encouraged me to put in writing how I want to be treated in the event I can't speak for myself. The document directs my family and potential bedside staff in care versus comfort. I'd seen so many people tortured in the name of saving their life that making myself a Do Not Resuscitate was an easy and clear decision. It was surreal to sit in the parking lot of the law firm with a mask on as I scribbled my familiar "AC" initials next to "Comfort Care Only." It seemed like such an adult decision.

Signing the will caused me to look differently at my patients; I was considering my own quality of life. I longed to know how my patients ended up in the hospital and what could have been different. It was as if I could use that puzzle piece of knowledge to have an advantage in my own health.

Just about all our COVID patients were part of the high-risk population: the elderly and those with preexisting conditions making them more susceptible to infection. Luckily, I didn't fall into that demographic, but I was far from healthy. Much like our patients lying in the beds, my BMI read in the obese section.

I had always struggled with weight management, and my years working mostly night shifts had not helped my attempts at dieting. I did enjoy being active and thrived when on a fitness routine when I had the time and energy, but by this point in the pandemic I had given up most things I enjoyed: socializing, hiking, trying new foods, traveling, and any form of fitness. I was constantly tired and longed to take a break from night shifts. I had symptoms of depression and was struggling, and I needed a change. So, I submitted paperwork for a transfer to a day-shift position, eager to get regular sleep and put together some semblance of a life.

The switch to days was everything I needed it to be. I slept at night and was awake with the sun, a routine that allowed me to commit to early workouts and balanced meals throughout the day, both which helped improve my mental health. In my effort to rebuild a healthy lifestyle, I stopped drinking alcohol and started focusing on bettering myself. I also committed to refusing overtime work to give my body a break.

Returning to day shifts during the pandemic was the relief I needed it to be. Due to the nature of treatment, every single one of our patients was intubated and sedated, and all were receiving the same therapies. The circus that days used to be now had the feel of night shifts, running on skeleton crews and having people avoid us at all costs. Work became repetitive, and though we had fewer staff available, our ability to come together as a team was profound. We helped each other in all aspects of patient care and held on for hope as best we could.

With my new daytime routine I had more energy, plus a desire to find an "out" away from the constant critical care and death. I wasn't ready to leave my peers, but I knew I couldn't do this job full time for much longer. I'd been worn down prior to COVID, and I had reached the point where I didn't have it in me to stay at the bedside forever. So, I applied for an aesthetics course to be a nurse injector, an idea I had toyed with for years. I took courses in my off time and found a part-time Botox position to grow my skill. I was getting healthy and finding the silver lining in the frontlines of this war. Life felt as normal as it could for a little while.

19. Spilled Balsamic
January 2021

By the turn of the new year, I could feel the strain of the past one weighing on me. We were finishing up our second wave of COVID, and everyone was in a state of pure exhaustion. There were no longer friendly hellos in the hallways. And being mid-pandemic meant no vacations or weekend getaways; there was no way to rest, check out, or be taken care of. By this point, hospital staff were still working forty-plus hours. Nothing had changed.

Meanwhile, community support had died down, conversations were focused on the vaccine, and the term "health-care heroes" had become old news. Families were becoming demanding and mean, no one was getting better, and what hospital staff still filled the hallways was feeling deflated from the deaths, and worse, the burden of keeping people alive so inhumanely.

I was becoming angry and disagreed with how some health-care workers were acting. They snickered at eligible patients who had chosen not to get vaccinated. The general consensus was: "If you don't get the shot to save your own life, why should I be here fighting for it now?" I saw no difference. We were a hospital, weren't we? We didn't turn away people for not going to dialysis or not taking their blood pressure medications. Was this all that much different?

Pressure was mounting to get the vaccine. It hadn't yet been mandated, but talk was nonstop about who would be getting it first and whether there would be enough for everyone. On top of the vaccine spectacle was the fact that for nearly a year by this point we had been caring for these patients without success. We had not changed our protocols or care in any way that was significant, and patients were remaining intubated long after the two-week limit previously set by the entire US medical community.

Instead of accepting the fate we had witnessed of so many since the beginning of COVID, we didn't withdraw care. Prior to the pandemic, it had been rare to keep patients intubated for more than two weeks due to the effects of prolonged intubation. Sick patients who weren't responding to treatments would have been encouraged to die with dignity. For whatever reason, doctors now steered clear of these conversations as we kept bodies alive, dependent on machines to breathe and reliant on people who had no heart left to care for their needs or to be their voice.

There was no relief and no support for the frontlines. New York had stopped cheering for us. Ted, a trusted nursing friend who had been caring for souls longer than I had been alive, who was three-parts New Yorker mixed with one-part healing guru, could feel my emptying spirit. I asked him questions a child would ask a wise owl: Why are we arguing about the vaccine? Why aren't people getting better? Why are we causing these patients to suffer so long? Why can't we allow family to at least be with their dying loved ones? Why is all of this still reliant on nursing? How am I supposed to survive this? He hugged me tight and put me in contact with his wife, a spiritual director, who he hoped could offer me guidance.

We met, and it was surreal to sit across from her in a local park, as I hadn't been with anyone in public like this in months. I almost felt like we might get in trouble for meeting, but I didn't care. I needed support and someone to tell me I wasn't crazy for having the feelings of hopelessness and despair consuming me.

Rachel's smile was kind and her approach soft. She listened with compassion and related to me when she could, acknowledging how tough it must be working the frontlines. It was the first time I was able to connect my growing fatigue for caring for people with the massive toll it was taking on my heart. I felt full to the brim with pain, frustration, and the paralyzing feeling of not being able to help. I finally expressed that the large number of deaths was wearing on me. Rachel reminded me of some breathing techniques, encouraged me to keep journaling, and arranged to meet me again the following week. For the first time in months I felt a glimmer of hope. It was a relief to release some of the pain I'd been bottling up.

We were reminded every day there were even more people in the ER waiting for one of our unavailable rooms, yet not a single patient was improving enough to be discharged from the ICU to a lower level of care; they weren't dying quickly enough to empty the beds either.

All other floors of the hospital were full of patients who required critical attention, but there were no open beds available in any intensive care unit for hundreds of miles. The pandemic caused us to cut corners, make do, and look at people who needed help only to tell them there were people worse off than they were and this was the best we could offer.

Between working my new second job at a med spa and the relentless toll of COVID, I felt like a walking zombie most days. Then, after the emotional meeting with Rachel, I was drained of everything I had in me, but I was feeling cautiously hopeful.

In this delicate state, I arrived home with my truck full of groceries and began unloading bags. While picking up the last bag, I was flooded by the sweetish bitter smell of balsamic vinegar. I lingered in the tangy notes for a moment before realizing the bottle had broken in the backseat and had soaked into the carpet.

I stared at the mess. Gently, I put the bag back in its place, felt every glimmer of hope I acquired during my meeting with Rachel bleed out of my body, then sat down on the garage floor and glared into the backseat of my truck. I wanted to scream, cry, shatter the bottle, then curl into a ball and sleep forever. I didn't have the energy to do anything. Tears cascaded down my cheeks as I sat in silence.

Thoughts about wasted money and the time and energy it was going to take to clean up the mess raced through my mind. I looked at the groceries in defeat; I realized I no longer had time to food prep for my shift starting in hours. The hospital was sucking the life out of me, and I needed a break. I needed to care for myself. I was exhausted and depleted. I didn't have time for this mess. My hope was gone, and I cried for the first time in months in utter helplessness over my bottle of spilled balsamic.

Rumors about the vaccine, relentless working hours, and our inability to make a significant impact poisoned my soul. I could feel everyone's stress and fear. I felt for my patients, lying lifeless in beds like lab rats, and for their families who mourned their absence while holding on to shreds of false hope. My heart broke with them and for them. It broke for the family members who were sick during this time and couldn't visit, and for the endless people who would not get to say goodbye to their loved ones. And it broke for my coworkers who were just as weary as I was. There was no time to process the sadness, however.

It didn't matter how much I tried, my demeanor was limited to a halfhearted smile that easily turned to disgust. In mere moments, I would break down in tears or enter a rant about staffing ratios and other issues in health care. I was volatile and ready to be triggered like in a game of Operation. Thankfully, I was able to unleash during my meetings with Rachel.

She listened to me talk about my Aries tendencies and coordinated our meetings with the moon. She offered encouragement, telling me that I was doing a good job and making a difference even if I couldn't feel it. I wasn't expecting her to fix me, but I was hoping meeting with her would help me to find the spark that had gone out inside me. In talking about the Universe and the yin and yang of life, I recognized there was hope somewhere on the horizon. I just had to survive this time. Rachel gently suggested that I start journaling again as an outlet to release my "pressure valves," so I did. Writing has always been a way for me to let go of pain and confusion.

Everyone at work was as ragged and run down as I was, and we all had permanent indents on our faces from the PPE and discoloration from living inside a mask for fourteen hours a day. Our spirits were low, and our laughter only came at ironic moments, not joyful ones. We had become numb to death and fear.

Instead of the occasional glass of wine after work, it became my routine to finish an entire bottle and then break into a second. And I wasn't the only one. Under different circumstances, my coworkers and I would have requested a table for twelve at a local restaurant, drinking them out of liquor while loudly discussing all the horrific things we had seen. Our now-blackened sense of humor would be making light of things most people couldn't fathom. But we were still in the pandemic, so gatherings of more than two people weren't allowed. Besides, we were all too exhausted to gather . . . or laugh anymore.

20. Horoscopes and Crystals
July 2005 – Current Day

My spiritual journey started when I was a teenager and had an obsession with astrology. I longed to understand what it meant when someone on the movie screen said, "That's because you're a Scorpio." The bizarre terms—*Libra, Capricorn, Taurus*—sounded like aristocracy, and I wanted in.

Fortune-telling, palm reading, and stargazing all seemed magical to me. In fact, the only reason I picked up a newspaper in my twenties was to read my horoscope. *Will I stumble across the love of my life today? Should I play the lottery?* But rarely did the Universe deliver such gifts; rather, I read warnings about tough encounters ahead or needing to manage the many volatile emotions of an Aries, and I was always reminded to be open to opportunities. But no matter what the horoscope said, I'd feel better after reading it. It was as if to say, "Well, now that I know what the Universe has in store for me, I can continue business as usual." It's such a silly thought that just thirty words some psychic-turned-writer whipped up to pay the bills can change someone's day. "Look, if my horoscope tells me not to buy a car today, guess who's not buying a car today? This girl." To me, nothing in life was predictable or the way it should be. A "your guess is as good as mine" approach is one I had adopted well.

When there was downtime on a night shift, the nurses would pull up the local paper on the computer, first to read all the want ads to see the odd things people would write, then to read a horoscope. It became a fun and playful counter to the black-and-white definitive world of medicine. Science and all its rational answers left little room to play with the unanswered or "what else is out there?" mentality. There was always a chance for a miracle or a sudden catastrophe.

By COVID times, I had gained enough knowledge in the field of astrology to offer astrological analyses of coworkers. I even went so far as to justify patients' erratic behavior by citing their birthdate and astrological sign. The dark days of COVID had me leaning heavily on spiritual resources. I dove headfirst into learning as much as I could about astrology and started frequenting the local metaphysical shops for tarot readings and crystals. Life was lonely, the world was silent, and pain was everywhere in my reality. If a pink rock in my pocket helped me love myself and other people a little more, then I was on board for the "woo-woo-ness" of it all. To me, it really didn't feel much different from intubating someone and leaving them to lie there for weeks on end with the hope things were going to turn around for them. The crystals and sage bundles gave me hope.

In my time away from the hospital, I practiced reading tarot cards and learning more about my own tendencies as an Aries sun, Leo rising with my Virgo moon. On full moons I wrote out all the things I wanted to release—past loves, bad habits, people I needed to forgive—and sat outside with my crystals as they recharged, releasing all the negativity I was desperate to see gone. When the new moon occurred a couple weeks later, I recharged and added a new routine and a wish to the powers-that-be that COVID would end soon.

I've always been accepting of the notion "everything happens for a reason." It's the only way I can justify having such a hard life. The anger I had toward my abusive childhood was too much to carry around, and I hated when people told me it would make me stronger. "Strong" was something I had locked down. I was traveling the country alone and making new friends in every fresh city; I was unafraid to venture out into the unknown. I was an ICU nurse who could pick up and fit in anywhere, one who could handle my own and be of service to a new unit. I knew my stuff as well as I could and thrived on taking care of those who weren't able to take care of themselves. But even with all I had been through, the strain of nursing through COVID had crushed my spirit.

21. Boiling Point
March 2021

Things were settling into a more stable routine. Finally, not everyone admitted to the ICU was COVID positive; in fact, we were able to separate our ICUs into one for COVID patients and one for anyone else requiring critical attention. It was a welcomed break from the hopelessness of COVID we were drowning in.

It was about this time, a year into the pandemic, we were informed administration would begin making daily rounds. We all groaned. Our manager told us they were coming around to help us and give us tools we needed. We rolled our eyes, some stormed out, and all asked how *they* were going to help.

There were additional forms in our charting we needed to fill out and new ways to score patients for everything from COVID-screening to fall risks. Every time the hospital delivered a new way to "score" something it meant there were more safety measures and protocols to implement. One more wristband to bedazzle the arms of our sedated patients. In written form it all sounded rather helpful, but it meant more paperwork for people who were already at their max workload.

No new resources or better staffing came with the additional boxes hospital execs checked off to make them feel like they were quantifying and addressing problems. It all just meant more work for the nurses, which inevitably meant even less time caring for the patients who needed us at their bedside. And now we were tending to more than just our sedated COVID patients. But administration smiled their pathetic grins and said headline-worthy phrases of "We can do this!" and "You're doing great!"

We were all tattered and defeated, and I had, quite frankly, lost hope in the system. Our once-ambitious attitudes had been beaten to a pulp, leaving a dried-out lemon rind where there had been bountiful life. The term *compassion fatigue* was meandering through conversations like a secret, and we all spoke about it on a global level. We rarely ever admitted defeat or held a mirror up to ourselves.

But I knew my ability to tolerate the strain of expectations, lack of support, and complete disregard for patients—not to mention the nursing staff—was limited. Every day I had to challenge myself to report to work. Every day I felt like I added fifty pounds of emotional baggage to my existing luggage I proverbially dragged into the hospital. Every day I came closer to screaming at the top of my lungs: "This isn't right! What we're doing isn't right!" but I bit my lip and tried to stay focused on the insurmountable task at hand—patient care.

For the past year we had been giving the same medications and following the same protocols, all for the same results. Anytime a nurse suggested trying something different, we were shut down. Words like *Ivermectin* became cringeworthy when suggested as alternative treatments. Doctors sternly told families over the phone there were no other options. It didn't take a rocket scientist to look around and realize what we were doing wasn't working. But why wasn't anyone trying anything different? Why weren't we throwing everything we had at patients and families who wanted a different outcome than death? At the very least, why weren't we letting family members in to be with their dying loved ones? Or clergy in to anoint and pray for them? It was infuriating. I felt utterly helpless for going through the same motions that would lead to the same results.

No longer jumping in to help, I instead busied myself in patient rooms. I avoided talking with patients' families at all costs. I had no emotional capacity to empathize, and my ability to break down disease and death into simple terms was gone. We all had an expiration date, and I couldn't fight for one life over another anymore.

I also steered clear of conversations with colleagues. When I did engage, I went into full-blown rants about how we were killing ourselves and no one cared. I'd rattle off the signs and symptoms of compassion fatigue (which we were all experiencing) and wave my hands in the air with hope a genie would fall from the sky and ease the burden. My rants became so passionate I couldn't tell the difference between exhaustion and rage. I felt as though any request might send me on a spree of flipping tables and patient beds, unplugging ventilators, and breaking windows. My attitude was foul, and my friends became irritable with my frequent rants and the anger spewing from every pore of my body.

We were through the second wave of the pandemic when the "suits" returned to our halls, walking through our unit in their N95 masks, gloves, and dress clothes that would hinder them if they had any legitimate reason to jump in and help out. But they were not there to help. With clipboards in hand, they sauntered around the unit in search of things to write down, complain about, tell us to improve upon, and remind us what we were doing wasn't enough—what we had been doing for the past twelve months wasn't enough.

Tensions were high among the nurses, and a palpable energy radiated through our scrubs. Not one of us rushed to hide our water bottles or turn off the music, nor did we try to hide our computers on wheels with saline flushes stuffed in the side bins. We continued as we had for the past year, managing as best we could for the dying people in our care. The tension must have been felt by the suits, as no one said anything to correct us or offer help. They simply jotted notes on their clipboards and carried on out of the unit. The nurses had given up on trying to impress anyone who had gotten to stay home since the beginning of COVID and were just now showing up to set tight margins again, margins that hadn't made sense in the first place and rules they exclaimed were for our "own good." But we were done letting the elites tell us how to live and function in crisis, especially when no one had shown up in the trenches of it. The inspections came at random for weeks, but we didn't change our routines.

I am sunshine and sparkles most days, beaming ear to ear with a grin that seemingly sings, "Life is wonderful, everything is perfect." It's not that I feel that way, mind you, it's just my resting happy face. Some people look miserable; I annoyingly always look cheerful. So, when my mood and energy shift and my unhappy side comes out, it's unpleasant and usually a shock to those around me.

Considering the amount of positivity I can exude on a good day, it *is* shocking when the negative monster comes snarling out. Born a fiery little redhead and an Aries to boot is a good-enough justification for my emotionally charged outbursts fueled with rage and pain.

Working the frontlines during COVID sucked out every ounce of joy and positivity I had. I tried to stay even-tempered when families asked me the same twenty questions over and over again with the belief I had an extra half hour to chat with them. Meanwhile, patients needed their hands held and their heads stroked but were lucky to have even been cleaned up from the soil they were lying in. The inability to effectively comfort was rotting away at my soul. My routinely chipper outlook came with sarcasm and outbursts of frustration at a system that clearly wasn't working. And with each suit perusing through the unit looking for fault, my blood boiled hotter and hotter. *We have lives to save; we don't have time to play your games.*

On top of the personal rage welling up inside me, I felt defensive of the patients behind the closed doors the suits avoided. I wanted to tackle these pristine, vaccinated humans, rip off their masks, and push them into the sickest patients' rooms, those who were choking on the tubes shoved down their throats to breathe. I wanted to put them in with the stench of stool, blood, and sweat that didn't disappear no matter how many times we bathed the patient. I wanted them to stand as vulnerable and helpless as we had stood while staring at a body being kept alive by a machine. I wanted them to look at the pressure sores on their faces from lying face down for eighteen hours. I wanted them to try and answer the family's unending questions we didn't have the answers to. I wanted to see them suffer the same way they were making the patients suffer—and, inevitably, the only people left standing to care for them.

Fortunately, I didn't have the energy to engage, so I ignored them as best I could and certainly didn't rush to make things perfect in their presence. I dared anyone to come near me and question why my water bottle was out or why I had an extra Fentanyl bag in my pocket: *Because the pharmacy cannot make them as quickly as we're going through them, Karen, and my next bag is about to run out in ten minutes, but I have a blood sugar I need to get, and I haven't charted a damn thing, but I had time to get this bag a few minutes ago for when the current one runs out.*

The Goody Two-shoes in me desperately wanted to follow the rules and do things by the book—individually checking out each med, verifying with a second nurse, reviewing the order for titration parameters before giving the choking patient an extra dose to ease the coughing—but there was no time for it, and it ate away at me to rush through saving lives. But that was the nature of the game.

We had been warned we would have daily evaluations at the patients' bedsides from a team of staff made up of mostly administration. I was on edge, ready to fight, and wanted to hear the ways they thought we could do better.

The time came for our bedside rounds. Our scrub-wearing manager accompanied the well-dressed team as they moved from room to room posed to make notes on their clipboards and tell the nurses how they could be doing better. We were given time slots for their visit, as if the ICU or any part of the hospital works on a routine schedule.

We stuffed away our sarcasm, put our heads down, and placed our water bottles and snacks out of sight. We tried our damnedest to fill out their forms, have the correct wristbands on our sedated patients, and make sure the signage outside the rooms was to their liking. Before long, it was 2:00 p.m. and my turn for rounds. The morning had consisted of a steady stream of problems needing resolving per usual with the addition of the new tasks.

I hadn't yet taken a lunch break when I looked up and saw several bodies walking toward me. Their fake smiles caused my teeth to clench, and I closed my eyes and reminded myself they thought they were helping. I answered every question with a short response, and if something wasn't to their liking, I simply replied, "Well, we're doing the best we can" with a forced smile. They nodded their heads and marked things on their clipboards before thanking me for my time. As they walked on to the next nurse who emanated the same emotions of irritation and faked pleasantry, one woman hung back and waited for me to pay attention to her.

"I was just wondering if you were aware of our nail policy?" she asked, tiptoeing with caution while pointing the end of her pen to my manicured nails. My home life had been falling apart and the only form of self-care I'd had the energy to keep doing was getting my nails done. For one hour every two weeks, I relaxed and allowed someone else to care for me. Having acrylic nails was against hospital policy, but so were the IV poles in the hallways, the extension cords running into patient rooms, and the staffing ratios they let us suffer through. My nails were the only thing I felt I had any control over. That, and the added support kept my nails from bending and breaking with every patient I turned and each medication package I opened. They were a built-in tool and the one last shred of self-care I was performing.

"I am," I said with the largest fake smile and sweetest voice I could manage. "Thank you," I replied, ending the conversation.

One round of administrative evaluations was all it took for me to beg my manager for a week off. I would have to take it without pay, but I had reached my max and was ready to snap. We were falling apart, losing ourselves, barely managing to maintain our sanity, and that woman had wanted to remind me I was not allowed to feel human! I wanted to explode like a grenade and take the entire building down with me.

Unfortunately, the break didn't help me at all; the only thing I thought about was work. I felt guilty I had stepped away while others didn't have the option to. I dreaded returning to the hospital.

By the time the third wave of COVID kicked in, the clipboards disappeared, leaving us to fend for ourselves. Zoom videos of encouragement from our CEO, sitting safely at home, began. They were pathetic attempts to try and dress our emotional wounds by telling us we were heroes. But we had no time to placate the false support—we had lives to save, people to take care of, and families to comfort. By then we knew who was on our side and who was riding the coattails of our unwanted heroism.

Administration was nowhere to be found in the times when we needed them most. Chief Nursing Officers (CNOs) didn't put on scrubs and jump in next to us; administration didn't serve us meals. Instead, our communities and local churches brought truckloads of food to the entrances of our hospital and stood under tents feeding our tired bodies. Those were the souls that kept us going. Thus, when the suits wanted to regain their position behind a desk, we scoffed at them and continued business as usual.

22. Back Injury Day
May 2021

I had at least showered that day. After more than a year of working the frontlines during COVID, my daily routine had dwindled from a robust morning ritual to ensuring my face was washed and teeth brushed. It was the most I could muster energy for anymore.

Showering had moved to an after-work event due to contamination, and I only showered after shifts at the hospital. I was sleeping until the very last moment so had just enough time to piece myself together with my less-than-stellar beauty routine before the eight-minute drive to work spent in angst about what nightmare was ahead. My once-peppy spirit and early arrival to set up report sheets and greet the day were replaced by a troll of a nurse ready to bolt out the door at any moment. The light inside me had dimmed, and there wasn't much left to shine. All that was left was a broken nurse who walked in for shifts with her head down, just on time, trying to keep every last minute of life not dependent on this place her own, trying to muster all her energy to face another day, a day of pure exhaustion and unbearable moments, even if no one died.

Driving to work, I found solace in the monotonous tune playing somewhere in the background. I no longer listened to pump-up sessions with inspiring podcasters or hype-up music; I enjoyed the quiet while trying my best to stonewall the memories of the previous day's shift and fighting off the anxiety of what the current day would bring. Empty, quiet, and growing feeble—I was beyond the reach of self-help and new morning routines. It took all the energy I had just to make it into work, so *how was I supposed to care for sick and dying people again today?*

I pulled into the parking garage, welcoming the darkness like a last hug before going off to battle. The ground was sprinkled with masks run over so many times they appeared to be part of the asphalt. Heaps of trash overflowed from trash cans that hadn't been emptied in weeks, leaving a lingering stench. I navigated around cones placed at the start of isolation. All the life once illuminated had turned to ash, leaving everything in a gray fog. Time had somehow stood still.

I sat there, unwilling to move. "Positive energy in, hold . . . sigh . . . and negative energy out. You got this. Four more shifts. That's it. Just four more shifts, then you get time off." I breathed in and gave myself a much-needed pep talk. "Come on, Ash. You got this. You can do this. This is what you were born for. It's just work. You're just a nurse."

Seeing others exit their cars in the same worn-out slump reminded me I wasn't the only one suffering and inspired me to turn the key and kill the engine.

"Four more shifts. I can do this," I muttered as I walked through the garage and put my mask around my ears to cover my face. I kept my head down. I couldn't afford to talk to anyone—I had no energy to give. I just had to get into work so I could get the day over with.

We traveled individually in a single line toward the sliding glass doors of the ER, ready to have our temperatures taken. The line slowed then opened up on the other side of the doors. Once again, there was no one to check temperatures. I guess no one cared if we were sick or not. I sauntered off to the ICU with all the gusto of Eeyore.

"I can survive this," I mumbled as the familiar slide of my badge triggered the beep of the badge reader and I heard the unlocking of doors echo as if inside a castle. *Maybe today won't be so bad.*

Lately, every shift seemed worse than the last. The first year of the pandemic we'd rallied together and worked with inadequate protective equipment, policies that changed daily, fewer support staff, more hours, and the same unknowing the rest of the world had—but we needed to show up and try to save those at risk of taking their last breath inside the hospital walls. It was difficult and intense and utterly draining. But we showed up, day after day, shift after shift. The problem wasn't COVID itself, it was that we were already running on empty after doing this work for so long.

The problems during COVID were not new to health care, they were just magnified: not enough support and not enough staff, all of whom were overworked, undervalued, and detached from their own loved ones due to the strain their hearts were burdened with. Stacy's familiar warning—"There's a reason we work in shifts"—had me hopeful those of us on the frontlines would eventually get a break. But no break came. We just persevered through hell, and what did we have to show for it? Nothing. Death and nothingness. Lost lives, distraught families, no resolution. At least before COVID we would occasionally see people recover, so we felt like we were making a difference then. Hope was highlighted among the loss. But not anymore. It felt like we were harvesting dead bodies. We all knew these patients weren't going to survive, but we continued to intubate and continued to try to be hopeful for our patients.

"You're in ACT today," the charge nurse said with a frown. She knew I didn't want to go to our step-down unit; she didn't want me to go either. And it wasn't that we had a surplus of nurses, it was that another unit needed the body (my body) more than the ICU did. My shoulders slumped and I hung my head in defeat. Being a float required extra energy I didn't have in me to muster up anymore. I turned around and trudged out the double doors toward the elevators.

I could just leave right now. The negative thought came without warning, and shame washed over me as I stepped into the empty elevator. I cursed myself for not being able to find positivity anymore. My upbeat self-talk had been replaced by survival phrases that did little to change my attitude, but they at least seemed to keep me in check enough to function and hopefully survive my last four shifts.

I arrived in the unit just as the huddle ended, so I went to a desk to print off report sheets. The last few moments before seeking out whom to get reports from had become some of the hardest moments I'd had to overcome. They were the last possible moments I could justify dropping my papers and running as fast and as far away as I could.

I wanted to run from the responsibility, the dreadful cycle of illness and death, the low staffing, and the shortage of supplies. I wanted to bolt down the hallways of patients who required much more help than we collectively had to give them; away from the burned-out, tattered, and war-torn doctors and nurses; from the managers who couldn't hold it together for their units anymore; from the respiratory therapists who didn't get the credit they deserved; and from the techs who had lost their ability to manage not just twelve, but now upward of thirty patients alone. *This is my last moment to escape everything I cannot fix.* But I stayed. I took a deep breath and forced a smile. *Four more shifts.*

I made it through reports on all four patients, thankful none of them were COVID positive so I didn't have to deal with PPE. One check in my favor. As I logged in to start prioritizing tasks for the day, I received a notification that blood was ready for one of my patients. The night-shift nurse hadn't mentioned blood, so I quickly reviewed charts and found a slew of STAT orders, from a PICC line to blood to CT scans, for a patient reported as stable. Sigh. I got up and went to her room. I hated this part of the job.

I needed to inform her about the new orders from a doctor who hadn't even seen her yet. Nurses are often put in a predicament where they're responsible for telling patients just enough to worry them but without details. In the fast-paced world of medicine, it's also our duty to see the next series of steps through. We can't give patients enough time to process information, and in the hurry-up-and-wait culture of medicine, there is no time for comforting.

It's not that I minded delivering bad news. I actually found a lot of reward in it *when* I had the time and availability to sit with patients to answer questions and comfort them. But I was forced to deliver this news and then run to get the blood I'd need started before she was taken for her scan. There wasn't time for pleasantries or feelings. There hadn't been for a long time.

I think most of us truly enjoyed caring for people and making someone's day, week, life slightly better, and that's why we stayed through it all. It's a blind obedience to the service of the well-being and healing of society. Luckily, ten years of nursing had taught me a few things.

I briefed the patient on all the new events since I'd seen her twenty minutes prior, including the NPO part, meaning she couldn't have anything to eat or drink. I mustered together the best smile I could and held her arm while looking her in the eyes. "It's all going to be okay. This is just standard procedure. Nothing to worry about. I do have to get a new IV in you and get some blood hanging, so I'll be bustling in and out of your room here, and some things are going to happen pretty quickly. Don't worry, you're in good hands."

While I reassured her everything was standard, I cursed myself for lying. It was a little more aggressive than just a standard GI bleed workup, and clearly her doctor wanted to get things done. She was to have an emergent scope, a procedure no one, not one single doctor, had come to talk to her about, and now they were calling for her STAT.

I closed my eyes, took a deep breath, and reminded myself I only had four more days of working like this, four more days of decisions being made last minute without communication, four more days of me explaining things I shouldn't be explaining to a patient so the physician can stay as far away from their care as possible, four more days of scared patients being brave for their spouses who are clueless as to how sick they really are, four more days of incessant call bells and the never-ending ringing phone, four more days I wouldn't get to eat a lunch or use the restroom when I needed to, four more days of everyone's attitude secondary to the pure disgust for the system we so ironically call "health care." I rolled my eyes and jumped up to prepare my patient for her surprise procedure.

A transporter showed up to take her to CT, and I was relieved to have time to see my other patients. I spent the time during her absence catching up on tasks for everyone else. Then, when my patient arrived back to the floor without notice, I scrambled to find staff who could help transfer her. We gathered around, all of us knowing the drill. I led the count.

"On three. One . . . two . . . three!" We all grunted while moving the patient from the stretcher to the bed. I stepped back and down off the bed like I had a hundred times before, although this time, the floor wasn't there. I felt the inevitable momentary stuckness of falling until my body was jostled to a standing position. Stars flooded my eyes as pain shot up the back of my leg. I winced, threw my head back, and inhaled sharply. I was hoping if I didn't exhale, it wouldn't be that bad. I stood with my head tilted back for a moment recalling what had happened. I internally scolded myself: *Why didn't you lower the bed more? Why didn't you call for more help?*

I exhaled slowly, allowing the notification of sensation to reach my brain, then dropped my attention to my back. What initially felt like an electrical shock had dulled to a "stubbed toe" sensation in my right hip joint. *I can work with that.* I opened my eyes and bent to focus on my patient. *Nope!* I straightened back up automatically. *Bending is not going to be an option.*

The other staff members were already on their way out the door. The wince I held in, the scream I smothered, the gasp that didn't get to escape in the nanosecond between injury and continuing care escaped in a breathy, tearful thank you to the nurses for their assistance.

"You good?" my charge nurse asked, pausing momentarily.

I knew she would help me if I asked, but she was needed by so many other people. I didn't know whether I was okay, but I was low on the priority list of thirty-plus patients and visitors, and the doctors and ancillary staff needed me to do my job. I nodded even though a disappointed voice echoed in my head telling me otherwise. I hobbled around for the next two hours in an attempt to finish all the tasks for my delicate patients.

Whether I was okay or not was irrelevant in this reality. If I wasn't okay, then I needed to report to the charge, give up my four patients, and proceed to the emergency department for scanning. And then there had better be a real injury or it would be a waste of resources. I was in pain, but I decided I could manage.

On my return to my sweet patient's bedside, I could see she was weary from a long day of testing and emergent decisions. I hoped she could see my eyes smiling above my mask and recognized how genuinely I wanted to be there for her. We'd been through too much together that day to quit then. So, I tried to put her at ease as I hobbled around the room while reconnecting her to the monitor and taking her vital signs.

The pain continually shot up the back of my leg, and I had moments of bending and twisting when I thought I might not be able to stand upright again. I moved cautiously yet efficiently as possible to finish my shift. The rest of the day was a blur, but I know it was difficult due to my extreme pain.

Charting on my four patients, certain I hadn't gotten all my tasks done, caused me to stay two hours past the end of my shift. I then made the careless decision to forgo reporting the injury in lieu of getting home in one piece. The only thing I wanted after this awful day was to get home without crashing. I knew I wouldn't pass a field sobriety test if asked to because of my exhaustion. So, driven by instinct, I headed toward the safety of my home and a hot shower to ease the physical and emotional pain racking my body.

Three more shifts, I reminded myself as I reached for the lunchbox I'd never gotten to open. I limped down the hallway, moving at a turtle's pace, magnetically drawn to any way out of the hospital but too war torn to move with excitement for the end of the day. It was as if I were in the last scenes of a horror film where the hero, bloodied and injured, crawled out from the depths of a hell only she and her slain enemy would ever experience. That's exactly how leaving the hospital felt most days.

Every motion took maximum effort, every step a step closer to refuge. I staggered to my truck and winced as I lifted my right leg to climb in. I gingerly settled into the driver's seat, exhaling through the pain. That same monotonous tune from over fourteen hours prior drifted from the speakers at a low volume, but the thought of any noise invading what little space was left in my brain was triggering.

"Shut up!" I said, punching the power button. I was on a sharp edge from pain and exhaustion, worried about the patient I didn't want to leave but couldn't bear to stay for, the patient who I now feared wasn't in the most capable hands. I was angry at the staffing and how we had all been run to the bone that day, like we were every day. I was angry at the other patients who needed things and at the doctors who thought we were their personal servants. I was angry I'd been floated and had injured myself, angry I wasn't tougher and that I now felt terrified my walls were crumbling. I couldn't believe I found so much negativity in a career I'd loved so wholeheartedly not that long ago.

I drove in silence down the dark roads without anticipating turns or stops, being guided by a survival instinct I didn't have to tune in to thinking about. I had both hands on the wheel as I stared straight ahead with one goal in mind: just get home. Watching the garage door open was like anticipating a welcoming hug, a sign of sanctuary and comfort. As I drove in, the sound of the door closing behind me signaled the end of the day, the closing of the castle gates. The final click rang out as the chain settled into place, and the garage door became a protective wall embracing me. *I was home.*

I wanted to fall on the floor and sleep for weeks, but I stayed focused on making it to the shower. I kicked off my shoes in the garage and replaced them with the slippers I'd left there that morning. Typically, I'd rip off all my clothes and throw them in the laundry room (the result of years of being cloaked in MRSA and C. diff had developed good at-home habits, yet COVID felt even dirtier). That night, though, I went straight for the wine rack. Without thinking, I methodically grabbed the corkscrew, opened the bottle in three fluid motions, and felt like my own personal cup was being replenished as the sound of glugs filled my wine glass with a sea of deep burgundy. Tipping the glass back, I closed my eyes and relished the sweet taste of home. As I let the liquid linger on my tongue without any agenda, I reached for the bottle of ibuprofen.

I wearily climbed the stairs, one step at a time, dread overcoming me both physically and emotionally. Without realizing it, I had been holding my breath since the injury. Now, inside my house, I brought my attention to my body and felt not only the sensation of a pulled hamstring and an ache in my lower back but also the cold and heavy weight of emotion bubbling in my chest. Every inch of my body was tired.

I made the journey up the stairs, one hand holding my wine and the other grasping the railing. At the top I flicked on the light switch, set down my wine, and looked at myself in the mirror for the first time in hours. I was unrecognizable. I was still in my scrub cap, and the indents from the masks remained visible, a look I hadn't gotten used to in the past year and half. It made me feel inhuman, cut off from the world, more ready for work and less ready to hold the hand of someone who needed me. I noticed my glasses were dirty even though I'd worn goggles overtop them. I pulled them off and was left with the red indentations of where they'd sat on the bridge of my nose all day. Additionally, my ears were tender from holding the weight of two masks, glasses, and goggles. I reached for my scrub cap, pulled it off, and grabbed my wine glass in preparation for viewing what was left of me, the wreck of a human I was about to face. My hair was matted and messy, there was a bright red line across my forehead, and though the lines on my cheeks were lighter, they were still visible. My face looked scarred and beaten.

The release from the constraint of the cap, mask, and glasses caused a frenzied sensation. I pulled at my scrubs as if they were burning my skin. I wanted to be free. *Get me out of these!* I scrambled to strip out of a uniform that felt life-threatening. My whole body began crying before the emotions actually hit. I'd been breathing heavily since I started climbing the stairs. I knew there was a hurricane of emotion brewing, but I just needed to make it into the shower. Every movement caused strain on my screaming leg and back. I moved slowly and methodically, stopping every few moments to gather strength and compose myself. My breaths were becoming shorter and faster, and I had begun to whimper.

I turned the nozzle and water gushed from the faucet and then the shower head. The spray ignited a deeper cry from my chest. Turning the knob, I ensured the water was hot enough to distract me from the pain in my heart and in my back. I wanted to feel it burn me. I took a long swig of wine and a deep breath before delving into the turmoil about to explode from my rumbling chest.

With a shaking hand, I set my wine on the counter and climbed into the shower, slowly relying on my right leg for balance as I lifted my left leg into the tub. *It hurts. It hurts so much.* I leaned my forehead against the cold tile and stood for a moment as the hot water hit my back. My breath trembled, and I began to sob. At first, it was a cry of defeat and disappointment. *How am I here?* But soon, my cries turned to wails as waves of pain and frustration spewed from my body in noises unrecognizable to me. With every sharp inhale, I unlocked a vault of emotion stored within. I sobbed for feeling weak and injured. I cried for the patient I couldn't do more for. I cried for the patient in the air vac that was landing even though we had no bed available to save someone else. I sobbed for nurses who were falling apart like I was, and I cried for the system that had pushed me to this point. The whole day replayed in my mind. There I was, alone in a career sucking the life out of me, without hope, without relief, without the know-how of what to do next. Helpless, hopeless, I sobbed.

Suddenly the realization I had to return the next day hit me and I cried harder, then screamed. There was no way I could do that day again. My soul ached as I wondered where I was going to find the strength and courage to show up again. *How can I fight for someone else's life when I can't even fight for my own?* The exhaustion had won, and I no longer even had the energy to mourn. The harsh reality of needing to do it all over again and again sobered me.

When my cries softened to breathy hiccups and my shoulders slumped completely forward, I finished showering with as much gusto as wet spaghetti. Initially, my intention had been to clean the stink off from the day and stretch my lower back under the hot water, but I was only able to half-heartedly wash my body and wet my hair. When finished, I stood numb under the scolding water, not thinking or moving, just merely trying to be alive. Hobbling out of the shower, I could smell the sweet, clean scent of myself and a wave of comfort found me as I climbed into bed. I curled into a tight little ball and suffocated myself in the blankets. *I have nothing left to give this day. I am done. Today, I am done.*

Before I knew it, my alarm sounded. I reached for my phone and was instantly reminded of the pain in my leg and back. *Oh. Right.* I flashed back to the evening before, still feeling the heaviness in my chest and puffiness in my eyes. There is something redeeming about waking up after a hard cry, but I did not feel redeemed this time. *Only three more shifts.* I slowly and robotically got out of bed and prepared for another day on the frontlines. I didn't allow myself to think about the day that passed, the day ahead, or the tightness in my leg—I just donned my battle gear.

23. Resentment
May 2021

Never did I think I'd be afraid of sneezing or dread putting on pants so much. It felt like my hips had turned to lead and locked in a contorted position, causing my muscles to scream out in sharp pain.

I was diagnosed with a pars fracture and acute hip dysplasia. The causing factor was the weight of every ounce of pain I was carrying from the health-care industry. I certainly didn't know it then, and I could not have described it as anything other than a twelve out of ten for pain through whimpering cries (yes, I am *that* patient).

I was a ticking time bomb of pain and rage. Every part of me oozed the despair, death, and abuse built up in me throughout the past ten years in the industry, an industry where nurses often serve as the filter between life and death and humanity proudly wears us as a shield even when the rest of the world is kept safe. I felt like a sponge for grief that was suddenly too full to absorb any more. I broke in every way that a human spirit can break.

Thankfully, I ended my contract and took time off. The injury had interrupted the much-needed vacation I'd longed for, making the thought of returning to the bedside any time soon unbearable.

It's not that I stopped wanting to care for people. It was heartbreaking, actually—I still wanted to be helping at the bedside. I wanted to be strong enough to stand by my peers who were burned out, overworked, and undervalued. In a way I can only explain as hollowness, it felt like all the love and drive I had to save lives and care for people had been drained from my being like a gas tank marker plummeting far below the lowest notch.

Along with the anger I held for the situation was my shame for leaving the bedside. I was just as good as any other nurse who was standing strong—why couldn't I endure more? Why wasn't I stronger? Why did I break? I was born to be a nurse and work at the bedside. I could handle it, I could see hope in the moments of hopelessness, and I could be a comfort when someone needed a warm blanket or a hand to hold. I could save a human life and respect their soul within.

My passion has always been to help people, to care for and nurture human life. But truth be told, I couldn't handle it anymore. I could no longer find positivity in the hopeless moments, I had no energy to advocate, I couldn't find an extra shred of time to devote to care, and I could no longer do the job that requires many more hands. The physical demands of the job had always been there, but the emotional toll it had been placing on my soul was too much to bear.

No longer could I help absorb the pain of my patients. I had no space for the aches of the general public. I could not listen to the mundane complaints about the lives of my friends and family. In fact, I was crumbling under the pain of my own careless injury, which to no surprise occurred on the clock and while caring for patients. No wonder I fell apart under the pressure of being understaffed and overworked while in the middle of a pandemic.

24. Withering Flower
May 2021

Saying goodbye felt different this time. After years of practice due to relocating every three to six months, I had become a pro at saying "see ya later" and meaning it. I thought I had forever to travel, make friends, and keep adventuring, all while helping save lives. But this time around I didn't feel as if I would be returning. I'd told everyone at work I needed a break and would be back soon in the same way I had been at the end of every travel assignment. But I didn't know then that for the next six months I wouldn't be able to even drive past a hospital, let alone return to work at one. I was burned out, having panic attacks, and feeling depressed and confused about the purpose of life. I was dumbfounded by the ways in which I had abused my body, soul, and spirit in trying to save lives through a pandemic not meant to have survivors. I was buried under heartache and disappointment—not to mention the physical pain from an injury that had left me nearly immobile. The only thing I'd ever known for fact was that I'd wanted to be a nurse. Years later, I wasn't sure if I had made a difference. I wasn't even sure whether I was capable of being a nurse anymore, as I could barely care for myself.

After my injury, I had to go back to the basics of self-care. Showers became an "as needed" task (PRN in nursing lingo), as did eating. My friends called but I'd silenced my phone. When they texted, I replied with a few words to keep them from asking too many questions. I kept my blackout curtains drawn all day, casting shadows on my unmade bed. How could I possibly show up for others? How could I bathe someone else when I didn't have the heart or energy to bathe myself? And my job as an ICU nurse required so much more than bathing patients. Besides, it took all my energy to prepare for the one-day-a-week injection job I had taken on months prior.

I didn't have the mental capacity to tackle the many things needing to be calculated and managed in a critical setting—for twelve-and-a-half hours . . . potentially without a break. And I certainly didn't have the capacity to anticipate and note minor changes indicating a decline in a patient's status. I couldn't do all the work of my *own* job in addition to that of others because of understaffing and too few resources. I most definitely wouldn't be able to talk to families for very long. My ability to be optimistic, kind, and compassionate was so drained, I may just say, "Your husband is dying. The sooner you realize this the sooner we can stop torturing his body and soul in the hopes of just a few more days on this earth, and the sooner you can move on with your life."

THAT is not the nurse I am. I am mortified I had become so drained and weak that my ability to filter reality through a lens of love, kindness, compassion, empathy, and understanding had evaporated from my soul. I realized I no longer belonged at the bedside. I'd lost hope in caring for people. I had to finally consider that my role as an

ICU nurse was no longer the right fit for me. Potentially, my role as a nurse in any form was no longer right for me. But how had I ended up at this point?

In retrospect, I could see the roller-coaster ride that required balancing my career and lifestyle and how it had gotten me so brashly to this humbling point. Burnout. Compassion fatigue. Depression. Pure exhaustion. I do believe, however, I'd lived my nursing career like I live my life: fast, impulsively, intensely, which ultimately led me to burnout much quicker than my peers. And once I started reacclimating into society, I realized the feelings I'd been experiencing more than a year ago were now symptoms the nurses whose sides I had to leave were facing.

Obviously, the breaking point for me was COVID, but my burnout started long before that. I'd been hopeful the huge numbers of lost lives, plus witnessing how far nurses are willing to push themselves for humanity, would have together been enough to allow for more bedside resources and support, thus changing the system. That has not happened. It appears as though the powers-that-be have seen how hard they can whip a workhorse and get results, so they have not let up. Unfortunately, this workhorse is dead tired. It's bizarre for me to think I dedicated sixteen years to nursing and now I'm no longer able to care for another human life and can barely care for myself. Teachers, first responders, military workers—the people who serve our communities while risking their lives and well-being—know this feeling all too well.

1

2

25. Nursing Myself
June – July 2021

Kinesthetic tape and Arnica gel soon became my best friends. The pain was very present but my excitement for freedom was greater, so while decked out in the finest muscle tape and jean shorts, I hobbled out on adventures and appointments that filled my calendar for the first few days I was finally free from the constraints of the hospital. I was anxious for the time off to dive into holistic courses and see friends. COVID restraints were lessening, and I craved a new lease on life.

Taking 800 mg of ibuprofen every four to six hours isn't exactly ideal for your body, but it was the only thing I had for the pain. The few Vicodin pills I had left from an oral surgery and the muscle relaxers stored away for back flare-ups just made me sleep and didn't help my pain. In my nurse's brain, I could rationalize the injury, and anti-inflammatories were the most prescriptive medication I could justify. They just weren't helping much. So, I did everything in my nursing, holistically driven mind I could think of to do for myself: yoga, icing, crystals, and meditation. But intensity increased as my emotional ability to handle the distress from the pain waned. It didn't take long for the burst of energy I'd experienced over my newfound freedom to die out, leaving me limping around—exhausted, overextended, and burned out. The Universe wasn't going to let me get off that easily.

Meanwhile, money was going out three times faster than it was coming in, and my backup plans were dwindling in support. The thought of going into the hospital was answered with my very quick and hard "absolutely not." I would not show up to the ER and be a burden to the already overwhelmed staff. I would not make myself an additional problem in light of everything already happening; besides, I had a good idea of the course of action and refused to be dismissed with a prescription for narcotics and a list of specialists to see. I knew if I followed the normal health-care module, it wouldn't be long before a specialist would tell me my only option was surgery, and I wasn't willing to undergo that until every other option had been exhausted. I'd seen plenty of patients who'd had back surgery to know that one surgery is never enough. I refused to live my life like that starting at age thirty-four.

My body was out of alignment; I could feel it. I could feel the discs pinch, sending jolts of electric shock down my legs and causing my toes to go numb with every wrong move. My hips were angled like a seesaw, refusing to settle into a normal stride. My femur jammed into my hip socket like a prison shank. Every movement reminded me of how broken I was, but I didn't want to be silenced with narcotics and a "maybe this will work" surgery. A good doctor would recommend physical therapy before surgery, and I didn't need a $90 copay to tell me that's where I needed to start.

By week two I'd booked an appointment with a chiropractor who offered PT in the office as well as help from nurse practitioners. The pain and discomfort in my lower back and hips was so severe I couldn't sit during my consultation with the doctor, so I leaned against the wall while viewing the sixty-five-inch television screen displaying an image of my own skeleton. The light grays, blues, and whites illuminated the silhouette of a human spine and stood out against the contrast of the black backdrop.

I frequently take for granted my medical knowledge and forget that to many people, an x-ray is a cool picture rather than a key to ailments. Though I hadn't had much experience in reading for ortho exams, I could recognize the spinal column staggering up the center of the screen, bending and curving to the left and right like a topographical photo of a river. I remembered hearing rumors when I was younger that I may have scoliosis, but to see it so blatantly on the screen made me uncomfortable.

While I wasn't a triathlete, I took pride in believing I was taking decent care of my body. But there in high definition was proof my body was weak, unstable, and defective. The click of a computer mouse brought up a new image, one that focused on my hips. A red line with markings clearly highlighted the unevenness of them and noted the degree of difference in centimeters. The picture was obvious even without the red marking. I was in trouble.

The doctor explained the findings to me as I fought to get out of my nurse's brain and into one of a patient. I wished I weren't alone. I needed someone else there to process all the information for me. I needed someone to listen to the details so I could play the part of the patient. Holding back tears from pain and disappointment, I put my emotions aside and tried to listen.

I agreed to everything recommended: trigger point injections, eight weeks of PT, chiropractic adjustments, red light therapy, and ibuprofen that wouldn't completely destroy my stomach like the over-the-counter tabs I had been taking. I agreed to anything that would keep me out of the hospital and relieve some of my relentless pain. I was eager to be a pristine patient; I was hopeful I'd heal in the prescribed eight weeks.

Physical therapy and chiropractic adjustments seemed to help in the beginning. My positivity and willingness to heal came with my usual upbeat attitude and as much effort as I could possibly put into my home stretching sessions. For the first couple weeks I experienced small improvements, and I was hopeful that in two months tops this would all be a distant memory. I continued on as intentionally as I could, finding hope and positivity a little more forced than naturally inspiring.

Though my pain was lessening a bit, my mood was decaying and dragging down my will to push through with it. I hobbled by for a few weeks to save face for a family visit, spending just enough time to rejuvenate slightly before heading home to fall into a pit of despair. For months I felt like a shell of a human. The discomfort kept me from wanting to get out of bed or doing any type of self-care including showering and cleaning, and the last thing I had energy for was socializing. When I did go out it was awful, like watching Uncle Fester getting reacclimated to the Addams Family. At any moment, my attitude could turn sour from pain and I'd have a complete inability to be in public.

It seemed as though anything could send me into a hurricane of tears or a tsunami of negativity. The perky and positive Ashley everyone knew was replaced by a dark, cloudy, energy-suck of a tornado with no personality and a new talent for bitchiness. I was in constant pain, and the moment my mouth opened, disgust for the health-care system and the lack of concern for those working the frontlines and our patients poured out.

My energy was a roller coaster with pain riding in the lead car. Some days were better than others, and some days were downright unbearable. The pain kept me from having much "get up and go." Many days I just laid in bed until I absolutely needed a drink of water or more pain meds. Now, I've never been a fan of narcotics, and after handing them out like candy at work, I'd learned enough to know they would never actually fix the problem. So, I saved those couple pills for nights when I couldn't sleep or the pain was excruciating.

On days when I had PT, it took all the strength I had to put myself somewhat together, climb in and out of the truck, and limp my way into my appointment. Adding an extra stop such as the grocery store was not in the energy forecast, so I lived off Indian food delivery and spoonfuls of peanut butter.

The ideal patient I imagined becoming required a lot of energy. I was alone and barely able to make it to PT sessions, let alone find the drive to stay positive. The pain was debilitating and emotionally exhausting, and sometimes I would just start crying from being totally overwhelmed and feeling alone. The thought of having to change positions to get up for water was such a feat I would cry myself back to sleep so I would forget I was thirsty. I slept without caring whether I woke up, sometimes hoping I wouldn't. I didn't want to wake up and return to the reality that had become my life.

No one was around. No one came to check on me, nurse me, lay out my pain pills, or bring me water. For most of my life I'd been devoted to helping people heal, surrounded by caretakers, nurses, and caring friends, and suddenly no one was there to nurse me. We were in the midst of another COVID wave, and my nursing friends were drained from caring for others. Loneliness and disappointment were like salt to the proverbial and literal wound. I longed to have help.

COVID wasn't over, but my ability to survive its devastation was withering away.

26. Seeking Advice
November 2021

When I went to see Dr. Potter, I was a broken mess. The pain had been persistent for months and only seemed to be getting worse. I was working sporadically at the med spa, my emotions had fully taken over, and I was in a constant state of gloom.

When I realized no one was coming to save me, it became glaringly obvious I needed to save myself. I had been a miserable human to be around; my friends had no interest in dealing with me, plus they had their own challenges going on.

I felt completely broken. I no longer wanted to be a nurse. I no longer wanted to be alive. So, my decision to see a naturopath was an easy one when the alternative meant going to the same health-care system I was so wounded from. I wanted to do things naturally; I wanted to regulate my emotions and body and manage my pain in a way that wasn't so caustic, in a way that didn't cause numbed-out emotions, weight gain, brain fog, and gastric upset. I knew there were options outside what Western medicine had to offer.

I'd read an article in a local magazine about Dr. Potter's arrival in Tucson. It spoke of her approach to natural medicine and healing. I called the number listed and to my surprise she answered the phone. I immediately apologized for calling, insisting I could hang up and call back during business hours.

"I like to be available for my patients. How can I help you?" she asked in a comforting voice. I was awestruck. Here I was, a simple patient she didn't know, and she was already willing to help me in her off hours. Eager not to waste her valuable time, I told her about my depression and the pain I couldn't seem to escape. She seemed confident these were things that could be managed, and we arranged for an appointment later in the week.

I thought about canceling. Correction: I thought about just sleeping through it, too drained to interact. Reluctantly, I put on yoga pants and a tank top after having a crying fit over spilled toothpaste and the utter doom that followed.

Dr. Potter's office sat snug between furniture stores in a quaint shopping complex tucked in the middle of town. I walked into the sunlit waiting room where a cheerful face greeted me. The receptionist sat behind a simple desk, kitty-corner to the door. I kept a brave facade as I introduced myself, holding back a mountain of emotion. It was all I could do to communicate with another human. I sat in a chair in front of floor-to-ceiling windows overlooking a small patch of green grass sticking out against the brown desert background.

Tall and thin in professional dress and dangling earrings, Dr. Potter walked out with a bright smile. My arms longed to hug someone. I wanted to tell her how much I liked her earrings and how safe I felt there, but I couldn't communicate. Keeping my arms crossed tightly across my body, I trailed behind her down the hallway, my head hanging low. I followed her back to the office where we sat divided by a glass-top desk. She recounted our brief phone conversation as I nodded along in agreement, trying to hold back tears and trembling with anxiety.

Normally, I would be open about everything. As she asked questions about my sleeping habits and symptoms, I nodded my head, straining my cheeks into tightly pressed lips to avoid sobbing. I felt so broken and ashamed about the state I had allowed myself to get to. My injury felt like a weakness I'd been hiding from the world. I felt unloved, unwanted, uncared for.

I was embarrassed she knew I was on the verge of crying with every question she asked. Each response was slow as I searched for words and tried to regain composure before answering. Every question revealed more parts of me not okay. I had been disassociating from myself in order to stay alive, and I now realized it was somehow killing me more.

I told her I was a nurse, and the tears started to flow down my cheeks without the accompanying whimper of a cry. Sadness came in waves as I tightened every inch of my body in desperation to hold it together. I felt ashamed that I knew about health and wellness yet had let my nutrition and physical mobility slack off in the depths of my depression.

"Does it feel like your cat is on the ceiling?" Dr. Potter asked.

I gazed up at the ceiling tile in the corner of her office and pictured a cat with its claws dug into the cardboard-like texture, fur on end, hissing, feeling stuck and terrified to come down, not sure about what to do, not wanting to fall to its death, but too frightened to take a step in any direction to come down safely. Tears flowed down my cheeks as I nodded my head. This was exactly how I felt—frightened, stuck, hanging on for dear life. What kind of nurse had I become? Shouldn't I have been able to take care of myself?

"Well, we are going to get your cat off the ceiling, okay?"

She typed notes on her navy laptop as she spoke about what she had planned for me. I was to stop at the local Indian market to pick up some herbs for tea to accompany the supplements she would send home with me. She then made long strokes along her arm and explained how to dry brush. She could see the overwhelm in my eyes as I tried to take in this new information.

"Don't worry, I'll write it all down for you," she said, pointing to her laptop. She then walked me to the front of the office and pulled bottles of supplements off the shelves, and we booked a Bowen therapy session for the following week. Trembling, I gathered the bottles and dry brush, said a very pitiful thank you, and headed out the door.

Climbing into the safety of my car, I took a few deep breaths and tried to convince myself to make another stop. What I really wanted to do was go home, pull the blackout curtains, crawl back under the covers, and sleep until I wouldn't wake up anymore. But there was something about following the "doctor's orders" that made me pull up directions to the local health market. It was close by, and if I wanted to feel better, I had to do what she recommended.

Once at home, I placed the herbs in a pot and let the water boil while writing on the lids of the supplements. I set my new dry brush on the counter along with the oils. I finally felt like I had a plan. I was drained from the day but feeling ever so slightly optimistic.

Along with my new routine from Dr. Potter, I vowed to start making my bed and opening the curtains every morning again. They were small tasks, but I knew they were imperative to my healing journey. If she believed that I could get better, I guess I could too.

27. Finding God
December 2022

When I was thirteen, I swallowed every pill I could find in the cabinet, washed them down with as much rubbing alcohol as I could handle, then chugged peroxide to ensure something would work. But the karmic joke was on me that day when the peroxide bubbled up in my stomach and I vomited. I sobbed as I stood staring at multicolored pills covered in fizzy gastric slime. I was still alive and now terrified about getting in trouble for the mess I had made. I was sick over being so disconnected that others couldn't see my pain or the obvious signs of an attempted suicide, both of which made me feel even more invisible. The ache of survival felt like salt in the wound.

I suppose if I trace it back, this suicide attempt was one of the first obvious moments I remember contemplating the existence of God. At the time I did not see my surviving as some act of mercy, I just thought God was punishing me by keeping me alive. I had no other justification for my painful childhood, and at thirteen, I could not see beyond the confines of the loveless home I was living in to any kind of brighter future. At the time my family was heavily involved in a Pentecostal church, thanks to my step-grandmother.

"Have you ever seen those church cult things on TV where they dance around with snakes?" I'd tease. "Being Pentecostal is like that but without the snakes." Talking about our religion always felt more like a warning than an invitation to join. I thought it was weird and over the top; it was "existentially melodramatic" as MTV's Daria would have said in her slow, bored voice.

Testimonies are a large part of the born-again Christian faith and were given frequently by anyone who felt compelled to share. The testimonies members shared from the pulpit were dreadful, raw, and full of pain. As a teenager I was always so jolted by these stories of things I didn't need to hear. I think the elders believed it was scaring us away from premarital sex and drug addiction. For me, though, it made church feel dirty, as if it were only a place sinners went to. It made me feel like in order to find God, one had to have some really awful hardship occur in their life to be worthy. I had been through some insanely awful hardships already. I had seen the devastating effects of sin and addiction and had been on the losing side of child predators. *So why hadn't I been able to see God?*

When I decided to leave the church at sixteen and prove that good people could exist and not be Christian, it almost became a mission of mine to do good despite all the bad in the world. It was in my nature to be kind and compassionate. After living a childhood riddled with manipulation and having to gauge the emotions of every adult in the room prepared me to handle even the most difficult patients and impatient ICU doctors who snapped at every question.

But here I was at thirty-four years old having lost my passion for the only thing I knew: to be in service of others. I was crumbling under the distress of emotional and physical pain. Almost twenty years after turning my back on God, I now found myself asking *why* to anything out there that might exist. My house had become an altar to salt lamps and Zen prayer flags, Buddha statues and good luck charms, positive energy and Feng Shui. I was trying everything, but I didn't own a Bible. After admitting to myself that I had never actually read the Bible, though, I thought maybe before I made a hard judgment that perhaps I should at least own one.

I believed in the good in people, knew to my core that Mother Earth had a healing energy all her own, and frequented the local alternative stores for crystals and sage bundles. I sat underneath full moons, crying and begging the Universe to either take me from this miserable new existence or remove my physical and emotional pain. I journaled as much as I could bear seeing my emotions in written word, cried at every inconvenience, and leaned heavily on reading my tarot cards for a sign that life could and would get better. I said positive affirmations and begrudgingly started getting outside again.

I came across a Christian video on YouTube and found some inspiration in the pastor's message. He was young, hip, and digging right into the core of what I was going through: "If you feel like you are stuck and the devil is holding you back, you have got to put your faith in God knowing he is there for you." He clapped with every word he shouted.

I scoffed in agreement. *Yeah, no kidding the devil is knocking on my door.* I was doing everything I felt might help, but the last thing I had yet to try was actually showing up to the building I feared would cause me to combust on entrance. After seven months of hanging onto life by frayed strings, I found myself in a church just a few weeks shy of Christmas.

By this point everything I spoke about involved the Universe, from job opportunities to who I was seeing to my healing. I was sure everything was connected. I was desperate to find meaning in the struggle and was faithful to the belief that whatever journey I was on there were spirits there guiding me. I understood science and summed it up as a simple case of all humans, life, and earth being made up of cells and atoms and believed we were all connected spiritually. Going to church couldn't hurt, and I longed for community. I looked around and saw the joy on people's faces as they worshipped God in a safe space, with hands raised and singing off-key, all in the name of love for something greater than we can explain.

I don't believe you can serve in health care and not believe in a power beyond what we can know and understand. This is not to say that all health-care workers have faith or must be Christian; in fact, most I have met are not. But it's hard to look at the science, the patients, and the variables and not account for something else we can't control. So how is this field of medicine and presumably caring so removed from a guiding source of hope and light in this world?

I wouldn't be where I am without accepting Jesus into my heart, and I don't know whether anyone is more shocked than I am myself to hear these words. Losing myself in the care of others made me see there is so much more to life than what we are given at face value. My journey through one of the darkest and most helpless periods of my life revealed a relationship I have forever known was there but failed to recognize. My hope is to one day bring God and faith back into health care, to the patient bedside, where the only one who can heal the blind is the one we keep out the most.

28. Who's Gonna Flip Your Grandma?
May 12, 2022

I was a withering flower in the environment of bedside nursing. Removing myself from the health-care system was the only option I had. The problem was, I didn't know who else I was if not an ICU nurse. I had already tried my hand in a variety of positions, from Botox nurse to hospice nurse to recovery room nurse.

Luckily, I found a seemingly perfect nurse recruiter position that was remote. The job allowed me to work on self-care while not having lives reliant on me. At first, I was overjoyed to help my peers find travel nurse positions. The pandemic required more nurses to travel, and I knew firsthand the benefits traveling could offer. I also knew the bedside needed strong nurses, and if I couldn't be there to help, then I would help direct them.

Shortly after I started the new recruiter position, hospitals began pulling travel nurse contracts, leaving the pool of jobs barren almost overnight. Deflated, I attempted to reach out to nurses, begging them to do the same job for less money, the same job I could no longer show up to. I couldn't blame them for not wanting it.

I had to reach out to my manager for words of wisdom on how to get excited about selling these jobs to nurses. "You just aren't money hungry enough, Ash," he said. His words made my temperature rise. I wasn't there for their money (I mean I *was* so I could pay my bills), but these were nurses we were talking about. I couldn't fathom how we were throwing them to the wolves like raw meat. Instead of reaching for budget, I catered to my small team of six travelers, sending them cards and stickers—notes of encouragement for continuing to do the job so many of us had tapped out from.

"What are you guys doing for Nurses' Week?" I asked over a Teams meeting, seeking advice from the seniors on my team who had dozens of travelers and were faring well themselves after the COVID gold rush.

"Ha. It's been Nurses' Week for two years; they don't need anything else," our usually clever team lead and highest in sales said with a chuckle. I was speechless. I didn't know where to start; I wanted to let a rampage of defensiveness and compassion spew from every inch of my being. Instead, I emailed my boss a two weeks' notice that afternoon and applied for nursing jobs back in the ICU.

The anticipation for the day ahead had me wide awake at 2:38 a.m. I laid in bed and pretended I wasn't awake, trying not to acknowledge the excited energy coursing through my veins. *Veins! I love a good juicy vein, and I love sticking a needle in it. Man, I love being a nurse. I hope tomorrow makes a difference!*

I lulled myself back to sleep only to wake up three more times before my 5:50 a.m. alarm sounded. I surprisingly felt bright-eyed and bushy-tailed on this glorious day. I had set out my favorite pair of black scrubs and my Arizona State flag compression socks the night before. Dressing on that morning was both a celebration of the nurse that I had been and the change about to take place. It felt as if everyone in the world was putting on scrubs that morning in anticipation for the march in the capital.

I had a perma-smile plastered across my face from nervous excitement. "Today, we're going to make a difference!" recited over and over in my head as I stood in front of the floor-length wooden mirror donning my battle armor and mascara. I heard my brother moving across the hall and my heart filled knowing he was up earlier than he wanted to be to support his big sister by driving me to the metro station.

The night before we'd looked at the metro map and reviewed the different routes I could take to and from the city. The sixth-grade field trip I had taken to Washington, DC, twenty-five years prior hadn't left me with any memory of the city or how to navigate it, and although my brother and sister-in-law were more familiar with how to get into the city, they were just as much novices as I was for attending a rally or giving in-depth directions. My ignorant bliss and history of being able to figure things out in the moment have been a blessing and a stressful curse.

My brother and I listened to stand-up comedy and talked about people from high school while he drove the forty-five minutes in morning Beltway traffic, him sipping his coffee and me drinking my smoothie. Our time together was strangely comfortable in a way we had never experienced as children. It felt ritualistic, like something ordinary families do every morning; the simple things we could only dream about as kids. Like the dad he was becoming, he handed me a metro card from his center console, adding to the two his wife had given to me the night before. They wanted to make sure I was taken care of, and although they didn't know how much money was on the cards, they wanted to support me.

As my brother pulled up to the terminal of the metro station, I squealed when I saw two people (who were obviously tourists because of their nervous approach to the gate entry) holding signs and wearing backpacks—nurses! I just knew they were on their way to the rally, and I couldn't wait to meet people who were there for the same reason: to march on the capital to demand reforms to the health-care system. My brother handed me an umbrella and wished me good luck as I jumped out of the car eager for the adventure ahead.

The metro card machines are giant with a lot of information on them, and I had to take a breath to calm myself to read the directions. *You're a nurse; you have traveled the country by yourself and figured it out every step of the way. You got this. Focus.* I watched the pair as they headed off in front of me, unaware I was there to stand in solidarity with them. By the time I made it through the turnstile, they were gone, and I assumed they would get on a train ahead of me only to be a distant memory. The escalator delivered me to the platform and I walked toward the small crowd of people awaiting the train.

The couple and I were now standing closely together, so I asked, "Where are y'all traveling from?"

"South Carolina," one of them answered, her soft southern drawl melting like butter on a warm day. She smiled and both introduced themselves. We made small talk about the distance traveled for both parties and our excitement for what lay ahead before the yellow train came whizzing by us and screeched to a stop. We sat across the aisle from each other, but they soon drifted into their own worlds while staring out the window, back to being strangers.

I watched morning commuters participate in their rituals, climbing on and off the train almost instinctively. Then, while pulling out of our fifth stop, I saw women in scrubs carrying rolled up poster boards, and I wanted to bang on the windows to let them know I was there too! I wanted to cheer them on and hug them, grab their hands, and run as fast as we could into DC! But then the train pulled out of the station without them getting on. Wait! I wanted to yell at the conductor, "Those are our friends! We can't leave without them!" But the women didn't look worried, they were just waiting for the next train. Panic struck—was I on the wrong train? Was I supposed to get off? What if I missed the rally? What if I never made it to the march? I looked over at my seatmates and they seemed unmoved, so I pulled out my phone to look at the map my sister-in-law had sent.

Nope, I'm still going the right way. I had to calm my mind and remind myself that my brother had said any train could get me into the city. I rolled my shoulders, closed my eyes, took a deep breath, and coaxed myself into calming my nerves. As the stop for McPherson flashed on the neon sign, I gathered my backpack, stood up, and prepared to exit.

This platform was much busier than the others. Tons more people were moving in all different directions toward signs pointing this way and that. I looked around and saw my new friends standing next to me.

"We saw you getting off and you looked like you knew where you were going, so we followed you," one said with a sweet drawl. I smiled back, happy to have companions.

"Well, I don't really know where I'm going, but my sister-in-law gave me pretty good directions, so I'm sure we can figure it out." I looked at my phone and recited the next train we needed to catch. The pair helped find the signs and directions, and we were off to the next platform, the Silver Line. As we waited for our chariot, we talked about our nursing backgrounds and the excitement we shared for being in DC.

They were new nurses, three years shared time between them both: Mike in the ED and Adrianna in a cardiac step-down. I was overjoyed that young nurses were in DC to fight for our rights too! It wasn't just the complaints of the old and jaded; no, there were real things wrong and even the new nurses could see it. Hope beat in my chest.

On the second train we were accompanied by another nurse wearing a Nurses' March 2022 shirt. She was boisterous and chatty, and her excitement only fueled mine. I couldn't wait to meet more people. She pointed out her husband and son, exclaiming they were at the march to support us too, noting her husband was a respiratory therapist. We all waved in his direction and thanked him for everything he does in his job before he stood to exit the train at the next stop. Another moment of panic.

"Oh no, this is not the stop they told me to get off at." Worry washed over me, so I refocused and looked at my phone. I could follow the crowd or I could follow my plan, and my plan hadn't failed me yet.

"Good luck! Hopefully we'll see you there!" I shouted as our newest friend exited with her husband and son. Mike and Adrianna made a split-second decision to stay on the train after I reassured them I had clear directions and was planning to go on with or without them. Two stops later, the three of us got off the train in an even busier terminal.

At the top of the escalators to the street exit were two women wearing Nurses' March shirts directing us down the block toward the White House. The streets were busy, and large groups of people gathered on corners to cross. The city was bustling even more than the platforms below. There were people in Nurses' March shirts and scrubs everywhere. I smiled every step from the metro to the front of the White House, where I stood in silent awe over the crowd gathered around us. Everyone was there to fight for our patients. My heart swelled with pride for my profession.

The White House seemed insignificant at this moment. I wasn't there to see the White House; I was there to make a difference—to tell the world we were wounded and needed help, to shout out to everyone that we wanted to take care of their sick and dying. But could someone care about us? My new friends invited me to march with them and hung around while we all stared at the beautiful crowd, reading signs and pointing them out to one another.

"Patients over profits!"

"Safe staffing saves lives!"

They were quirky sayings written on old pizza boxes telling whoever would listen we'd had our fill of free pizza and were here to demand better.

"She is definitely a nurse manager of an ER somewhere," I jokingly said to Adrianna as a woman on a loudspeaker rallied the hundreds of nurses gathering together. We'd heard her before we saw her. Her short dark hair had a fresh buzz cut on the sides, while the top laid perfectly combed to one side. Her dark blue scrub bottoms accompanied her Nurses' March shirt over a white long-sleeved T. She held a pink microphone and called out to us, asking us what we wanted, reminding us we were there to demand better for our profession, and hyping the crowd to shout our call to arms! She traveled between groups, hyped up signs, and continued to encourage us to use our voices.

We spent two hours standing in front of the White House preparing to march to Audi Stadium. Anticipation grew and settled in a repetitive loop as we gathered our voices in chants of passion and advocacy, then calmed to a boring silence as we waited to march forward. A few times excitement washed over the crowd and everyone pushed toward 15th Street before being halted again. Rumors of waiting for the police to shut down the streets made their way through the crowd. Nurses, gathered in clusters, told war stories and laughed at things that would chill most people to the core.

Chants of "Who's gonna flip your grandma! Who's gonna flip your grandma!" broke out and was a fan favorite. It was funny, catchy, and true. We were shouting at the top of our lungs to anyone who would listen. Who *was* going to hold the hands of lonely grandmas when all the caring staff were forced away from the bedside?

"We want to care for you; help us, help you!"

"Cap ratios—not pay! Cap ratios—not pay!"

"What do we want? Better staffing! When do we want it? NOW!"

"Safe staffing saves lives! Safe staffing saves lives!"

By the time the mob began to march forward, we had a lot of practice with our chants. When the floodgates opened and the sea of people started to flow down Pennsylvania Avenue, cheers of hope and righteousness echoed. Chant after chant was initiated by one section or another, and we held our signs high while shouting about the injustices we weren't going to stand for any longer. Thousands of Hoka shoes (our nursing shoes of choice) walked the rally line. Children, husbands, and friends wore their T-shirts in solidarity. I remained with my newfound friends who had joined with others they knew. Our small group of nine stayed together, laughing and chanting. With me were young nurses who had spunk and energy and passion for change. My heart filled and cracked open knowing there were nurses who weren't as war torn as I was but still knew the dire conditions they'd had to endure in their short careers.

It's a sad day when nurses with less than two years' experience burn out to the point of losing hope. It's one thing to have a jaded human who has thousands of deaths under their belt and dozens of years' experience to be tapped out. But when that nurse who recently had a glimmer in their eye and a hope for nursing is feeling the heartbreak and pain from the sheer lack of ability to care not only for their patients but for themselves too, it's tragic. When most of a field is wearing down from a system that doesn't recognize the needs of the crumbling foundation, shouldn't we start considering something is wrong?

I assumed marches happened in the capital every single day and we were just another group marching and shouting for another cause. But there was desperation in our voices because we weren't shouting just for ourselves, we were shouting for our patients—the patients who belonged to the family of bystanders and people filming us from the fourteenth floor, the children witnessing their first rally in DC on a school field trip, and the construction workers who paused and watched us as we interrupted their jobs. We weren't here just for us, we were here for everyone. For anyone who might end up in a hospital bed or knew someone who had. For every single person who needed a compassionate hand to stroke their head or help navigate their medication list and save their life.

I thought our presence would make a difference. I waited with bated breath while I watched the evening news, then the nightly news, then the morning news the next day—nothing. There was no mention of the march in DC, no mention of the nurses who were crying out for help. We had been silenced. My hope plummeted as I flew back to Arizona to a career I was terrified to return to.

29. First Day Back
June 2022

It had been a year since I left the bedside. I had made significant strides in my healing; there were even days when I laughed, though not as often as I used to. I had an opportunity to return to a community hospital in town, and my finances were in need of replacing, so because I was feeling strong enough in health and stamina, I decided to try returning to the bedside.

I wanted to take all the tools I had been working on in my healing journey and put them to use in the hospital. I wanted to prove I was still a bedside nurse and the fault had been in me and not in the broken system. I ensured it was a day-shift schedule, knowing all too well my body would not be able to handle the stress of night shifts, even though the autonomy and pace of nights had some appeal for easing back into the environment. The seasonal thirteen-week contract allowed for light at the end of the tunnel and reminded me of a phrase my first recruiter had coached me with: "You can do anything for thirteen weeks."

I was going to intentionally return to nursing and wanted to make sure I took care of myself along the way. Ensuring nightly rest and keeping my circadian rhythm stable was a cornerstone of recovery. I left my schedule in the hands of the charge nurse with the simple request that I had every Sunday off.

Since stepping away from health care, I had found refuge in a local church and began attending faithfully. I planned to continue my current workout routine, to meal-prep healthy foods, meditate before and after work, and journal more about my experiences. As much as I could be, I was ready to give it a try back inside the hospital. I hoped God didn't mind the pink crystal I carried in my pocket to remind me to care for myself throughout the day.

On the day of my return, I woke too early, energy coursing through my veins. My body tossed and turned while I tried to convince my mind to fall back asleep. After an hour of redirecting my thoughts from the day ahead, I peeled myself out of bed and donned the workout clothes I'd neatly laid on the dresser. "Deep breaths, Ash."

Pins and needles pricked every inch of my body, and I fought the urge to chatter my teeth together and allow the energy to escape. Careful, concentrated movements accompanied slow deep breaths as I tried to focus on each motion my body performed. Downstairs, I sat on the couch and meditated in the dimly lit room. The world was still a night's dream outside. My mind coached me through breathing techniques I'd practiced so many times over the past year. *Breathe in for two, three, four. Hold for two, three, four . . .*

The soft alarm of the Alexa rang a digital tune notifying me the meditation was over. I raised my arms over my head, palms meeting at a point, then drew my arms down to form a triangle shape while my hands rested at my heart center. "The light in me honors the light and love in the world." Reaching for a familiar devotional, I opened to the first page and started to read. *Seeing Beautiful Again* was such a metaphor for the prior year that I couldn't help but return for the third time to read this book of inspiration and guidance.

Replacing my slippers with my shoes, a thought of Mr. Rogers crossed my mind and a smile creased my face. I stood, took another deep breath, and made intentional strides out the door. My morning walk was a familiar stroll past houses I'd made up stories for. The silence felt overwhelming; I was afraid to be left alone with my thoughts, so I allowed soft worship music to play through my headphones. Consciously and carefully, I savored every moment as I walked and took deep breaths. I redirected any thought that wandered off into anxiety about the day ahead back to the here and now, knowing I didn't need to be anywhere else other than walking around my cul-de-sac at 4:00 a.m. I had plenty of time; I was up a half hour earlier than I'd planned, and even my scheduled time left room for error.

"God, please be with me today as I return to the bedside. Please help me get through this day. I have no idea what to expect, but please help me to calm down and stand with me as you have been." Desperation oozed from my heart as I cried out, my voice trembling. "Breathe, Ash, just breathe. Focus on the palm trees silhouetted in the early morning dawn." I fixed my eyes on the trees as I walked past, trying to focus on anything except what was about to come.

Back at the house, I wanted to get moving, the natural reaction from a morning routine of years past, but due to the vast time I had in front of me and my roiling emotions, I kept my motions slow and intentional. There was no need to rush this morning, no need to feed the feeling of anxiety I had gathering at the nape of my neck.

I saw fear in my wide eyes as I looked in the mirror. The woman who loved to smile and goof off even when by myself was now terrified to be alone, terrified to think about what was coming next. So, I stopped thinking and started moving. I combed through my wet hair, put toner on a cotton swab, and applied mascara, all while swallowing back tears of anxiety. The sound of the hair dryer seemed to make the hairs on the back of my neck stand up. I wanted the comfort of a slow cup of coffee, but I was wired already and the energy from the blow dryer seemed to kick the anxiety hanging at the base of my skull into hyper drive. *I wish I could bottle some of this energy and save it for a rainy day.*

While making the left-hand turn into employee parking, I noticed a Mack truck pulling out from behind the hospital. I could see the familiar logo on its grill as the truck edged toward me. *If he runs me over, I wouldn't have to go in,* I thought, my biggest fear almost sounding like a wish. The red leather-bound binder of my will flashed through my head. At least I had everything in place. I made a last-minute decision to make a left in front of the truck, my body swinging along helplessly, not sure if I was rushing to survive or rushing to test fate and have the truck crush me. Relief then regret danced in my stomach as the truck blared its horn after barely missing my taillights. I made it. *Damn.* I was bathed in dread for returning to the hell I had escaped and yet hopeful to implement the new self-care tools I'd learned to rebuild my career. A feeling of nausea rolled over my body in waves. "Now you *have* to go inside."

I stepped behind the nurses' station and walked diligently toward the door I knew to be the breakroom. Not knowing where to start, I put my backpack down, grabbed an assignment paper, and left in search of my nurse orienteer.

"I'm with you today, dear," I said as Ted looked up at me quizzically. I'd forgotten I'd cut my hair short and the mask covering my mouth and nose left little room for recognition. A wave of sadness washed over me. He began a rehearsed welcome narrative before making eye contact with me and recognizing the familiar face before him. Ted wrapped me in a loving embrace as his sweet New York accent carved around his words.

"Oh, Ashley!" His excitement was more than I expected, and he held me in a long bear hug that nearly lifted me off the ground. Sitting down next to him with trembling hands, I tried to focus and login. After a brief report, I was feeling capable and ready to start morning care for my patients. The room felt familiar, the patient seemed familiar, the care was second nature. For a moment I felt like I had never left the bedside.

Just when I felt I might survive through lunch, we were asked to take on another patient because we were a team of strong nurses and there weren't enough nursing staff there. This immediately triggered stress in my chest, and I began to vent to Ted about the unfair staffing. We were already at max patients and now we were being asked to take on more because there were two of us.

After a forty-year nursing career, Ted has remained kind and somehow has not lost his ability to tolerate the system.

"You just do your best. You control what you can control and realize that health care is a business, Ashley. You cannot change health care or this hospital or this unit, and you may not even make a difference in someone's life today. But you show up and eventually you will." His words were encouraging but frustration raged in my chest.

"But this is wrong! We aren't helping anyone, no one cares about us, and this place feels like it's constantly on fire," I whined back like a little kid. Helpless, hopeless, and frustrated, I felt I'd made the wrong decision to return to the bedside. Later in the day, I was warned about the number of new grads on the unit and reminded that my skill and expertise would be needed. Waves of stress washed over me. *I can barely manage myself. I cannot manage anyone else right now.*

I can't do this, I thought over and over again on repeat in my heart. *This isn't right.* There was no support or safe staffing, there were minimal supplies, and the floors of patients' rooms were sticky with bodily fluids from who knows when. One of my patients was calmly and rationally coming out of alcohol detox, but I couldn't help but worry, what if that changed? If I had this many patients AND an actively belligerent and detoxing patient, my head might explode. It was too much to bear.

There was a code called in MRI and my stomach sank. Two other nurses responded as I sat stuck, shocked, traumatized. The old tingling sensation started at the base of my neck as if a sprinkler had just been turned on. I wanted to run out the door. I didn't want to be there anymore. I took a deep breath. Then another.

I was surprised by how easily being a nurse came back to me—caring for the patients without hesitation and using my old routine. Trying to avoid all new grads, I found structure in simply focusing on patient care. After all, that's what I was there for.

Not only did the charting and comradery flow like I hadn't been absent for a year, but it was also second nature for me to hit the Code Blue alarm and find the CPR pedal to lower the bed and do my first round of CPR since returning to the bedside. It occurred during my third shift and first shift without orienting with Ted. At 10 a.m. my ornery patient who had been arguing with me and calling me an imbecile all morning about a stool softener and enema had now vagaled down and flatlined.

"One, two, three, four . . ." I started compressions while looking up at the clock. *10:17 start of compressions.* I made a mental note as I waited for the team to show up. I could hear the code cart being wheeled from its perch, relief that people were on their way to help. Fortunately, this code was short lived, and the man's heart regained rhythm within the first round of CPR. Now on a vasopressor to support blood pressure, my step-down patient required the attention of an ICU assignment, though I continued to have four patients due to staffing.

Feistiness of the elderly can never be underestimated or even explained, and this eighty-something-year-old man awoke from CPR as if he had gained ten years. Not forgetting our previous argument about being NPO, an order given by doctors to not eat for various reasons, the patient continued to demand I make ordering him a meal a priority. His doctor was reluctant to start feeding this man whose heart had completely stopped while he was being evaluated for a bowel blockage less than an hour prior. The patient was furious and continued to verbally abuse me just moments after I'd saved his life.

It seemed like not just the act of nursing was coming back but so was the reminder we were not appreciated. Yes, I was definitely feeling that returning was a bad idea.

Five weeks into my return to the bedside and the thirteen-week contract I was counting down to the end of, the day I had been dreading most had come. The pandemic was deemed over, and it was my turn to float. For the past few weeks I had been able to dodge the float assignment due to senior staff pulling strings, buying me some time and sanity. They had made excuses or sent someone else in my place, knowing I wasn't ready to be thrown into the added stress. I kept the rants to a minimum, but it was hard to keep my mouth shut when all around me things didn't make sense.

"I'll go, but I'm not taking more than five patients," I threatened.

"You're gonna do fine, dear. Just do what you can and try to let the rest go." Ted gave me a bear hug and sent me off the unit with chocolates in hand.

It was absurd to ask for an orientation to the telemetry unit. I had been there before. It was absurd to management that I had gotten the two days I'd asked for in my interview to reacclimate to the bedside in the ICU. But I knew I needed time to adjust back into the routine. By this point, any extra nurse was needed to take a team of their own. We were but warm bodies to the system, warm bodies who could pass medications. Management and the likes had no concern for our skill set or knowledge base, only that we showed up and filled a void in their numbers. So, I was grateful for the orientation to ICU and, taking a deep breath, prepared myself for the familiar walk toward the telemetry unit with the knowledge that in just moments I would be thrown to the wolves.

Out on the telemetry floor, the energy buzzed incessantly. It was 7:00 a.m., and it felt like an ER in a downtown city. There were call bells and bed alarms ringing down both cross halls, and nursing computers on wheels sat strewn about the hallways unofficially marking a room where a nurse might be. There were no familiar faces left. There was no structure. It was every person for themself. I found my assignment, thankful to be starting with four patients and a new admit and unsure whether there were plans to give me a sixth. Five I felt I could handle.

What I wasn't expecting returning to the bedside was how high the acuity of the patients on the floor would stay after COVID. During the pandemic there were no other options but to put the least sick of the sick out on the floors with machines and needs floor nurses weren't used to. But post COVID it seemed like all the patients on the telemetry floor could justify a bed in ICU.

Of my five patients, one had liver failure and required continuous blood infusions. His family had just arrived from out of town and had a lot of questions. No doctor had spoken with them yet. I had a sweet seventy-something-old man with dementia and a new hip replacement who was in atrial fibrillation and needed monitoring. One of the call bells going off was his, and I soon learned he wanted to get out of bed frequently by himself with his brand-new hip, IV tubing connected. Luckily, his big blue eyes and giant smile kept me from being too annoyed. He immediately apologized in childlike innocence and attempted to climb back in bed all on his own. I also had an 8:00 a.m. scheduled bedside cardioversion I was supposed to be present for before discharging the patient home, opening a bed for an admit in the afternoon.

My fourth patient was a woman diagnosed with breast cancer. She was frail and fading, and I was surprised to find she was mistakenly put on double the normal dose of oxygen without the required humidity to keep her nose from drying out. She was quite uncomfortable and unable to advocate for herself or press her call bell. I took time helping her find some comfort, setting up her breakfast tray, and cleaning off her bedside table covered in trash. She looked like she had been forgotten about.

My last patient was a new admit for chest pain who was scheduled for a cardiac catheterization. I welcomed her to the unit and could feel her anxiety while she asked questions about the pending procedure; she had just received the news of the severity of the situation. I took as much time as I could to answer her questions, giving her a rundown of the procedure from start to finish and assuring her it was routine in an attempt to ease her fear. I wanted to answer every question in detail and let her cry, but there simply was no time for it.

Between getting my forgetful patient back to bed, hanging multiple units, cardioverting, discharging, admitting a new joint replacement patient, and wishing my patient well on her way to the cath lab, I only had time to check on my quiet lady down the hall a time or two. She was sitting alone in the dark and was refusing pain medications. I had no time to be with her.

Midmorning, a smiling new grad charge nurse introduced herself and handed me a patient report sheet. "You're getting this into room nine."

I forced a smile and closed my eyes, pausing to gather my composure. "I'm not taking another patient. Five is my max, and quite frankly, this assignment is rather heavy. I'm sorry. I'm not telling you no, I'm telling the hospital no. If management or administration gives you any pushback, just tell them to come directly to me." I coated every word with sugar to ensure I wasn't being defiant toward her. She was brave for taking a charge nurse role and just doing as she was told. She was merely the messenger. But I needed to put my foot down. Enough was enough.

The rest of the shift continued as I put out fire after fire, never truly feeling caught up, never truly being able to care for my patients, never truly being able to give any of them the care or attention they deserved. While walking back to the ICU unit an hour after my shift ended to gather the lunch I hadn't had time to enjoy again, I knew I needed to be done with the bedside. Sitting down at the desk before grabbing my bag to leave, I wrote a resignation notice. For the first time in nine years I canceled a contract. I was quitting nursing.

30. Medicine Under the Mango Tree
March 2023

By the time March 2023 rolled around, I was hanging onto my nursing license with a cold dead hand. I had already let my home state of Pennsylvania license lapse. Now, my coveted Arizona license was due for renewal, and I was stalling. I wasn't sure I wanted to be a nurse anymore. Every email notification made me consider whether I was willing to drop the RN and walk away from caring for people forever.

The past year had been a whirlwind of different nursing and non-nursing jobs with hope of finding something that sparked joy in my heart. I attempted to work from home, attempted a nine-to-five, even attempted to go back on contract in a local ICU. I'd tried nurse recruiting and dabbled in the world of aesthetics. None of it felt fulfilling, like I was making a difference, or was anything I could sustain for more than just a few months.

I felt inspired when my new church offered a venue for nurses to volunteer through a mobile clinic. I was eager to see what ways the church had found to offer care outside of the Western health-care model, but alas, they were also reliant on State regulations with no work-arounds. Everything in health care had to be done one way it seemed, and there was no possibility to just simply offer free help to people who needed it.

Volunteering had felt so wonderful and fulfilling until I felt like there was no good way to help. My hope for making an impact outside the realm of health care was squelched when I realized how much our hands were tied in the services we provided due to the State regulations.

I knew the regulating boards meant good and well in providing guidelines for safe patient care, but it was all too fresh for me and all still felt financially driven. I didn't want to be the link that guided someone into a health-care system only offering more medications for the sadness, pain, and grief engulfing the world.

Volunteering became a chore I dreaded as much as returning to the hospital. I was heartbroken that I had lost my ability to be a nurse. Every day I struggled to get out of bed and show up to care for people in whatever capacity I had agreed to that week. I continued attending prayer meetings and Bible studies, always praying for my passion in nursing to be restored.

I longed to care for humans and help them heal, bringing a smile to their face or a moment of peace during tribulation. But no matter what route I tried, I was left feeling unfulfilled, and unable to help in any meaningful way. I needed the paycheck to keep a roof over my head, but I couldn't physically bear being inside the health-care system. There was nothing I was certain of anymore except we were all eventually going to die, and I wanted to help people feel comfort while they were still alive.

On a last-minute whim, I booked a mission trip to the Dominican Republic with a group of strangers from my hometown. A friend had gone on the trip years prior and had returned with a renewed love for nursing. This inspired me to seek the opportunity to help outside the walls of America, hoping to redeem any scraps of love I had left for my dying passion.

I had no idea what was in store for me in the Dominican Republic; all I knew was if I couldn't find purpose in helping people with nothing, then perhaps my own purpose was gone.

Every moment in the Dominican Republic felt like a walk of faith. Because we didn't speak Spanish, we relied on local twenty-somethings who had learned English from watching MTV and *The Simpsons* to translate for us. We hiked into the jungled hills, past shacks and small villages of people who had little more than the clothes they were wearing to their name. Our fearless leaders had been coming to the DR for the past twelve years, bringing first aid supplies, simple medications like Tylenol and ibuprofen, and basic antibiotics, antifungals, and anti-parasitic medicines to the Dominican people. They also brought clean-water filters to communities removed from even the basic humanities of their own island's cities. We tried to educate people on hydration and basic symptom management through translators who had no medical knowledge. Day after day we rattled around in our van, driving up steep terrains and winding roads where we'd park and hike further into the overgrown jungle to the community center or church for each small village. We once set up a clinic under a mango tree for lack of any other space.

We welcomed the people who came to see us, smiled, and asked how we could help them. Most people had seen the team in previous years so knew we would bring resources and solutions. Some brought their children who had fungal infections on their scalps and protruding bellies. Others hoped for the simple relief ibuprofen could offer to the seventy-year-old man still doing hard labor or the postpartum mother with ongoing cramping. The people in these villages had some access to medical care if they were willing and able to travel to the cities and pay astronomical fees for medications we pay pennies to get. Offering real help to these people brought meaning to my soul, and though the nights were late and mornings early, I eagerly arose to go and serve daily.

One day I comforted a woman who came seeking something for her persistent back pain and broke into tears after I questioned her about the onset of her symptoms. She told me how for two months she had been the primary caretaker for her husband who had recently died. She looked at me as she spoke, telling me through the translator about how much she missed him and how hard it had been on her body to care for him. It had worsened the back pain she'd acquired years prior after caring for her dying mother.

The tears rolled from her eyes despite every swipe she made. I held her hands as I listened, staring into her heart and giving her space to grieve and hurt. When she finished her story and shrugged, she summed it all up with a request for ibuprofen so she could get back to work. I squeezed her hands and promised I wouldn't let her leave without something for the pain. Then I asked if I could hug her. She nodded her head, then let the tears fall without wiping them away. I stood and wrapped my arms around this grown woman who was sitting at an elementary school desk laying out her pain for someone who couldn't fix any of it but wanted to sit with her while she wept.

The other nurses continued to interview men and women, taking as much time as they needed with each. With warm smiles to make up for the language barrier, they handed out baggies of medications. I didn't see as many patients as the others that day. Instead, I sat with the widow who simply needed to be hugged and held. She had needed a loving caretaker to care for her, if even for just the short time she was at our clinic.

Inside a church with dirt floors and wooden pews, I drained an abscess on a man who'd been wounded at work. He had been passed around from doctor to doctor for a growing infection and simple antibiotics. His immediate smile of relief from the draining caused me to raise my tear-filled eyes to the sky and proclaim, "Dios es bueno!" *God is good.* I had been practicing saying the phrase with the translators during long bus rides, and at this moment the words rolled off my tongue as if I could say anything in Spanish.

Here I was able to help, my medical knowledge serving a community of people who needed education on clean water and infection management. They were beyond grateful for the samples of over-the-counter medications we brought along and the fungal soap we instructed the kids and parents alike to use. I educated them in simple terms about the detrimental effects of drinking the sodas and sugary drinks they were consuming instead of clean water, tiptoeing around the term diabetes, a diagnosis no one in this part of the world had the ability to afford or education to manage. I hugged moms, laughed with children, and shook the hands of old men who came seeking wound care and, sometimes, just a friendly smile. In the DR I could be the person I was put here to be: the loving, caring servant of the sick.

The week flew by, and I returned to Arizona feeling refreshed. I was still a nurse; I still had a heart for caretaking. I was just simply living in the wrong environment. My visit to the Dominican Republic proved helping others was still my passion, but I could no longer continue helping inside the walls of a system relying on its patients to stay sick to turn a profit. It was clear to me: I needed to get away from health care.

31. Let Them Eat Cake

Present Day

The health-care system is turning a blind eye to the well-being of their own employees and paying customers. Throwing pennies at the problem will no longer be enough to keep the beating hearts of the few souls left caring for our sick and dying. I want to jump up and shout, "REVOLT!" while leading every nurse in a march back into their hospital to demand conditions be different. But who has energy for that at this point?

But what if we start a little squeak of the battle cry right in the cozy and safe space of our hearts? "Revolt!" I say in the tiny, soft voice of the innocent child version of myself playing with a toy stethoscope. The freckles on my nose scrunch closer together as I give my best tough girl "grrr" for the belief I'll be strong one day.

That adorable little child inside of you is asking you to be brave too. But not against the health-care system, not against this seemingly endless pandemic, not against the political circus we're in or against ungrateful and abusive patients. I have no more energy to give to revolt against these systems. Heck, most days I can't drive home from work and spell my name at the same time.

I'm utterly drained, infuriated, and heartbroken. All the energy I have left I have to use to take care of myself or I'm afraid I will end up in the next hospital bed. So, I put on my most comfy sweatpants and hoodie, curl into a ball under the heaviest blanket I have, then let that little girl inside me holding her toy stethoscope whisper, "Revolt!"

Revolt against society telling you what you should be doing right now; revolt against your normal behavior of being super helpful and available; revolt against working endless overtime and feeling guilty about it; revolt against the minuscule pieces of cake being thrown your way as a hollow thanks for what you've had to endure for years.

I have dimmed my natural light and love for the care of others, something that took an act from God to intervene in. Don't let yourself get as lost as I have been. Revolt for the sake of yourself. There is power in numbers, and we frontline health-care workers are numerous in count and trusted most by our patients. We must truly take care of ourselves before we can take care of others.

What I have in my soul is unconditional love for humanity. No matter someone's race, creed, or driving factor in life—if someone is suffering, I want to help. Unfortunately, the unconditional love I have for others was something I lacked for myself.

The self-love and compassion I have gained through my healing journey is one that will benefit me for lifetimes to come. Removing the insulting factor, the health-care system, was the first but far from last step in this journey.

Having the ability to love myself while I was a miserable human, in pain and crumbling to pieces, was what saved me and brought me to an even stronger and unique place in this world, a place where I put the care of my own physical, emotional, and spiritual well-being first so I could help others along the journey.

Since there isn't medicine for burnout or a billing code for caring, I've had to learn to be my own nurse. I am learning I must first put on my own oxygen mask before I can help anyone else. Healing hasn't been pretty; in fact, it has been a disaster doing it alone. But somewhere in the middle of it all I have found myself, God, and strength I didn't know I had.

All the love and tender care I have delivered to patients in the last ten years and all the knowledge and skill I have gained are not for nothing. I have arrived at a beautiful place of independence and self-discovery where I can say with sincerity that we can all play a part in healing ourselves.

I am learning to intentionally move my body every day, stretching and strengthening my healing back. Instead of rushing to numb the pain away, I am learning to sit and listen to what my body is trying to tell me. By getting to and fixing the problem at the root, I am rebuilding a foundation of strength and wellness and rediscovering what health means to me. And I am learning that no matter what I know to be definite here on this earth, there is always space for faith. Science, in all its glory, always credits the margin of the unknown that can't be explained as the placebo effect. Some call these miracles. I think that mysterious unknown is exactly where we need to start exploring. What if we did make time and space for the possibility of power outside medicine and science?

Our patients deserve better. *We* deserve better. For the first time in my life I am not ashamed to stand up and say, "I deserve better." I refuse to take the abuse any longer, and I absolutely refuse to watch our patients suffer in a system providing neither healing nor care. If the best way to lead is by example, and people are looking to us for answers, why as nurses are we not sprinting toward health and wellness if for no other reason than for our patients? And if not for them, then why not for ourselves?

Acknowledgments

I would be nowhere without God's strength and direction.

To the patients who have allowed me to care for and advocate on your behalf: thank you for allowing me to love you.

To the nursing aides, RTs, and RNs who have stood tirelessly caring for people in their time of need, humanity needs more people like you. Please take care of yourselves first so we can continue to heal the wounds of this world together.

Carson, you have been the spark that reignited my passion for life. I hope you always know how capable you are. You are loved beyond belief, my little dinosaur!

Mary, thank you for being the very first person to believe in me and this story. Thank you for seeing an author inside this technologically challenged mess.

Freddy, thank you for making sure I eat more than girl dinner and reminding me to make time for self-care.

Alexander, thank you for the endless pep talks, rant sessions, and believing in this dream as much as I have from the start.

To my beta readers: thank you for understanding my passion for this project. Most of you stood next to me during a time in history we will never forget and continued to stick with me through the worst of it. This book would not be possible without you.

To Mr. Nic and Miss Wells who instilled a passion for the written word in my heart and helped me discover a way to express myself. Thank you for allowing me to turn in late homework.

To my family and friends in Pittsburgh who continue to love me even after I ran away to chase my dreams. Thank you for always welcoming me home.

Connie, thank you for giving me a shot in a big scary ICU. The family environment you encouraged allowed us new nurses to grow up safely and confidently.

To all the Sisters and senior staff on my home unit: you taught me how to be a bedside nurse and to love the human beyond the bed.

To the OG squad who has survived a decade of going in different directions: thank you for all the morning beers at Jacks and for not hating me for ruining Christmas when my patient removed his TDC.

Jake Dodds, thank you for writing a song that was the soundtrack to my healing. "She Goes to Work" played every time I sat to write.

To health-care heroes worldwide: I am brought to tears every time I think of how you ran to the frontlines without question, answering the call to serve and sacrificing your own life to help another.

To the staff still at the bedside: please put your own oxygen mask on first, make your self-care a priority, and don't allow the system to drain the passion you have for caring.

To every eager nursing student: please know your *why* and don't let anyone deter you from what you know to be right. Care for yourself first and let your cup runneth over with love for your patients.

Made in the USA
Las Vegas, NV
05 May 2024

89579294R00115